W9-BIP-100

"Anyone who believes that their biology is bound by time will be surprised by the groundbreaking science shared by Dr Hyman in this beautifully written book. Well researched, easy to understand, and inspiringly practical, *Young Forever* will be a game-changer for anyone who reads it, and for the world at large."

—Dr Uma Naidoo, author of *This Is Your Brain on Food*

"For too long healthcare has been *reactive*—providing care only after the wheels have fallen off the bus. Dr Hyman, the quintessential pioneer of functional medicine, shows us in *Young Forever* that the key to great healthcare is being *proactive*—detecting the warning signs of impending illness and intervening with lifestyle changes (and medications) as early as possible. This, with Dr Hyman's second piece of critical advice—fully believing your best days are still ahead of you—should help you truly enjoy and get the most out of your senior years!"

—Rudolph E. Tanzi, PhD, coauthor of *The Healing Self*

"In *Young Forever,* Dr Hyman generously provides a thorough and fascinating explanation of how your cells age, then he lays out a powerful set of tools you can use to slow your aging and rejuvenate your body and soul. Only the legendary Dr Mark Hyman could have written a book so broadly integrative and wise. This is a truly precious guide for vitality and healthy longevity!"

—Elissa Epel, PhD, coauthor of *The Telomere Effect*

"*Young Forever* is the ultimate guide to a long and thriving life. Dr Hyman synthesizes his decades of clinical expertise with a hoard of scientific literature to provide a clear, accessible, and holistic road map to a very optimistic future. The book covers the full spectrum of longevity tools, from foundational nutritional principles to cutting-edge advances on topics like peptides, glucose biosensors, and whole-body imaging. Reading it will help you better understand your body. You can start today towards optimal function and a bright future."

—Dr Casey Means, cofounder and chief medical officer of Levels Health

"*Young Forever* is an impressive guidebook to health and longevity."
— David A. Sinclair, PhD, author of *Lifespan*

"Dr Hyman expertly unpacks mountains of longevity research—the most exciting frontier in medical science today—to deliver an accessible and practical guidebook for living your longest and healthiest life."
— Nathan Price, PhD, chief scientific officer of Thorne HealthTech

"*Young Forever* implores you to contemplate the value of your years on earth and what you'd do with infinite health. Dr Hyman presents a radical new approach to aging, extending your health, and, more importantly, increasing the quality of your life. This book will teach you how to live better, for longer."
— Tony Robbins, coauthor of *Life Force*

"Dr Hyman is one of our leading functional medicine practitioners and teachers. In this vital new book, he integrates the latest science with his personal healing experience and decades of deep clinical insights, outlining a path toward growing older while staying young in body, mind, and spirit. An invigorating, illuminating, and innovative work that will enrich the lives of many."
— Dr Gabor Maté, author of *The Myth of Normal*

"An empowering guide to reversing the hallmarks of aging. *Young Forever* shows us that we already possess the tools we need to maintain a high quality of life, no matter our chronological age."
— Dr Sara Gottfried, author of *The Hormone Cure*

"Dr Hyman expertly distills the new research on aging into clear, actionable steps for reversing our biological age that anyone can implement in their daily lives. A must-read for everyone aspiring to a long, active life."
— Eric Schmidt, former CEO and chairman of Google

"*Young Forever* is a new key addition to my collection of books on longevity. In this genuinely life-changing book, Dr Hyman lays out the blueprint for living longer and healthier than many may have previously thought possible. A great read for all ages!"
—Dr Eric Verdin, president and CEO of the Buck Institute for Research on Aging

"Dr Hyman has once again seized on a trend and written an excellent book. This time it's longevity. *Young Forever* offers easily digestible science, legitimate advice for living longer, and Hyman's consummately readable style."   —Dan Buettner, author of *The Blue Zones*

"Anyone pursuing a long life of health and happiness must read this book. *Young Forever,* by my friend Dr Hyman, will change how you view aging. It will give you hope for living your best life for a very long time."
—Wim Hof, author of *The Wim Hof Method*

"Now more than ever it's clear aging is modifiable. Dr Hyman elegantly synthesizes recent scientific advances into actionable insights that can help us turn back the clock, improving our lives and those of our loved ones."
—David Furman, PhD, associate professor and director, AI platform, Buck Institute for Research on Aging

"If you want to apply the extraordinary recent discoveries as to how to prevent premature aging to your own life, there is no better book! This is a must-read for anyone who strives to create vibrant health throughout a century or more of living."
—Jeffrey S. Bland, PhD, author of *The Disease Delusion*

"Dr Hyman is one of the international leaders in functional medicine, and in this excellent book he combines his expertise, based on thirty years of clinical practice, with major recent discoveries in the longevity field to provide straightforward recommendations that will help readers live longer and healthier."
—Valter Longo, PhD, author of *The Longevity Diet*

YOUNG FOREVER

**THE SECRETS TO LIVING YOUR
LONGEST, HEALTHIEST LIFE**

Dr Mark Hyman

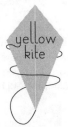

First published in Great Britain in 2023 by Yellow Kite
An imprint of Hodder & Stoughton
An Hachette UK company

3

A CIP catalogue record for this title is available from the British Library

Trade Paperback ISBN 978 1 399 71630 7
eBook ISBN 978 1 399 71631 4

Printed and bound in India by Manipal Technologies Limited

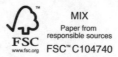

MIX
Paper from
responsible sources
FSC
www.fsc.org   FSC™ C104740

Yellow Kite
Hodder & Stoughton Ltd
Carmelite House
50 Victoria Embankment
London EC4Y 0DZ

*To the scientists, alchemists, dreamers, myth busters,
visionaries, and lovers who dare to push the limits of our
imagination and reinvent a better, healthier world for all of us*

Contents

PART III

THE YOUNG FOREVER PROGRAM

Do not go gentle into that good night . . .
Rage, rage against the dying of the light.

—DYLAN THOMAS

When you were born you cried and the whole world rejoiced. Live your
life in a way that when you die you rejoice and the whole world cries.

—NATIVE AMERICAN PRAYER

I'm not afraid of death, but I'm in no hurry to die. I have so much
I want to do first.

—STEPHEN HAWKING

Introduction

If you were asked if you wanted to live to be 120 years old, would you say yes? For most of us, the idea of living beyond our eighties is not appealing. Frailty, decrepitude, dependency, loss of mobility, pain, and disease seem the norm. But is that all inevitable? Is it possible to live into our nineties, hundreds, and beyond disease-free, active, and mentally sharp? The answer emerging from the field of longevity and aging research is a resounding yes! *Young Forever* explores that science but, more importantly, provides a clear road map and practical guide to incorporate the best of the science into a self-care plan that will help you live a healthy and long life.

However, there is a fundamental question you need to answer for yourself before diving into the revolutionary science that can extend both your health span (how many years you live in great health) and your life span (how many years you actually live).

What is your *why*? What matters to you? Why might you want to live to be 100, or even 150 or 200—which is not beyond current scientific possibility?

Much of our lives are spent building, making, and creating. Marriage, children, career, friends, a few vacations. But imagine that you arrive at sixty stronger, fitter, healthier, wiser, smarter, and more energetic than you were at forty? Imagine you have another 60 to 80 years left to live of a vibrant, highly engaged, functional life? What would you do? How would you spend your time? Who would you spend it with? I just turned sixty-three and am stronger and healthier and far wiser than I ever imagined I could be by applying the science of healthy aging to myself. As I look out over the horizon I can now give myself to those things that matter most to me—my family, my friends, teaching, and helping to bring the future of medicine and healing to the world.

For me the answer to *why* is simple: love and service. To meet myself, my friends, my family, and my work with love and to make the world just a little bit better before I die. To savor what I neglected in the busy time of building a family and career. To enjoy the gift of this life, the magic of being alive, the wonders of creation, the beauty and tenderness of other human beings. To serve and contribute to healing and more love in the world. To dance under the stars, to ride my bike around the world, to hike remote mountains, to learn new languages, to laugh and play and cry with those I love. To learn and grow and evolve my soul. That is my *why*. What is yours?

The Japanese, who are the longest-lived people in the world, have a concept called *ikigai,* or "the reason for being." In short, it's the state of four elements: what you love, what you are good at, what you can be paid for, and what the world needs. The science is clear—those who have more meaning and purpose in their lives live longer, regardless of their lifestyle.

We live in a world that is full of expectations and demands and struggle, and for many of us, when we finally reach our "golden years" we are spent, tired, and often sick. One in six Americans has a chronic disease, and according to the National Council on Aging, about *80 percent* of older adults have at least one chronic disease and 68 percent have at least two.[1] No wonder so few want to live to be more than 100 years old. Aging seems to bring inevitable dysfunction, disease, and death. Aging is scary.

But what if instead you could live to be 120 years old, go for a hike with your beloved, swim in a mountain pond, cook and eat a delicious meal, make love, and then just drift blissfully out of this life? That's how I would want to go. In fact, I am counting on it. But if that seems like a fantasy, it is only due to a failure of imagination. A failure to think about aging and disease in the light of the current science of human biology, a science that is disrupting all our concepts of health and disease.

Aging accelerates the risk of all chronic diseases—heart disease, cancer, diabetes, dementia, high blood pressure, autoimmune disease, and more. The truth is that what we see as "normal" aging is, in fact, *abnormal aging*. It is the result of myriad changes in our biology that are treatable. Aging is not considered a disease by most of medicine today. But what if we start approaching aging as a disease, and a treatable one at that? While American medicine has not embraced this idea, the World Health Organization (WHO) has officially recognized aging as a disease.[2]

But we are hampered by a medical paradigm that focuses downstream on symptoms and diagnoses, not upstream on causes and mechanisms. Remarkably the National Institute on Aging receives less than 10 percent of the National Institutes of Health budget—about $2.6 billion. And of that, only $260 million goes directly to aging research; the rest is spent on the downstream diseases of aging, like dementia, not on the mechanisms or underlying causes of aging.[3] Contrast that to the problems we are trying to solve. Our annual health care expenditures are about $4 trillion, most of which are for aging-related diseases. Does it make sense that we spend only 0.0065 percent of the cost of the diseases driving those trillions in spending on research into the actual *causes* of those diseases, while we spend the vast majority of research dollars on how to treat those downstream diseases? It's like mopping up the floor while the sink continues to run rather than turning off the faucet. Rather than study the root causes and underlying mechanisms of aging, we look for drugs to block abnormal processes and suppress symptoms. But even if we found ways to completely cure heart disease and cancer, we would add only five to seven years to our life span. Nowhere near the doubling of life span that occurred last century with sanitation, antibiotics, and vaccines. The cost savings of extending healthy years of life even 2.2 years would be enormous—$7 trillion over 50 years (or even more according to some researchers).[4] Now imagine if we could extend it 20 or 40 or 60 years. Yes, a society of sick and frail old people is expensive, but what if they weren't sick? What if they were healthy and strong and contributing to their families, communities, and societies?

There is a scientific revolution happening today that is forcing us to change our entire view of health and disease. It is a paradigm shift as big as the discovery that the Earth is not flat or that the sun doesn't revolve around that Earth.

This revolution is called functional medicine (also known as systems medicine or network medicine)—which looks at the body as an ecosystem, a web of complex interconnected networks and systems that regulate our biological functioning; systems that, when out of balance, drive dysfunction and disease. It turns our approach to diagnosing and treating disease upside down.

The flaw in our approach to treating disease is that we think all diseases of aging—from heart disease to cancer, dementia, diabetes, and more—are *different* and that we need to find *different* cures for each one. However, the truth is that largely, they are just manifestations of the same underlying changes in biology that occur with aging and are highly influenced and *modifiable* by our lifestyle and environment washing over our genes.

Modern medicine treats each individual disease as if it were a distinct entity separate from everything else that happens in the body. This is whack-a-mole medicine. We even have a word to describe how we think of these problems as separate. We call them *comorbidities*. A person can have high blood pressure, abnormal cholesterol, heart disease, diabetes, and cancer, and we treat all these as separate diseases, when in fact they are all just slightly different manifestations of the same underlying dysfunction in the body. Rather than asking why aging is the biggest risk factor for all these diseases, dwarfing smoking, obesity, and other "killers," we treat them all individually. It's upside down.

The exciting discoveries emerging from the field of aging research point to a radically new approach. Science is getting to the root cause of why we get sick and why aging is often accompanied by decline in function and decrepitude. If we understand the *why*—the root causes and the changes they trigger in our biology, in our interconnected web of molecules and cells and tissues—then we can transform our health and well-being and extend our lives, both our health span and our life span. By addressing what are often called the *hallmarks of aging*, we can prevent, treat, and even reverse most of those diseases without directly treating the disease. In *Young Forever* we will go even deeper and map out how to treat not only the hallmarks of aging but also the *underlying causes* of the hallmarks of aging.

This has been my life's work: studying and applying this new paradigm of medicine, functional medicine, to tens of thousands of patients over 30 years. Diving into the networks, excavating their biology for clues to the root causes of disease, investigating the upstream drivers of disease. I have deeply explored their genetics, microbiomes, immune function, hormones, mitochondria, detoxification systems, and structural systems—the network of interconnected systems that explains nearly all disease. It has given me a deep understanding of the weblike ecosystem of our biology and has helped millions of people around the world.

The beauty of this approach is that it is never too late to start. Yes, starting at birth or even before is better, but the research is clear: Making changes at any age, even seventy, eighty, or ninety, can create profound changes in health and longevity.

Personally, I am training to be the healthiest 100-year-old I can be. What does that look like? It might be slightly different for each of us, but I define it as being able to get up in the morning and do what my heart and soul want to do: climb a mountain, read a book, go helicopter skiing, surf, play tennis, make love, no matter what my age. I want to continue doing what brings me joy for the rest of my life. But I don't want preventable physical limitations to impede my ability to live life fully engaged, mentally sharp, and physically active. At sixty-three, I am in better shape than I was at forty. In fact, my biological age is forty-three years old. What I have learned over the last few decades is nothing short of revolutionary in helping me get biologically younger while I grow chronologically older. I want that for you too.

I have struggled with many health issues over the last 30 years, and through my own disease, pain, and suffering I have learned how to heal myself and so many of my patients. At thirty-two I had back surgery with complications that left me with a weak leg for the rest of my life. At thirty-six I developed chronic fatigue syndrome. For more than a decade I struggled with crippling fatigue, brain fog, digestive issues, muscle pain, and immune dysfunction—I had to find my way out by treating mercury toxicity, mold exposure, Lyme disease, autoimmune disease, and more. I learned how to heal my body using this new medical paradigm, addressing root causes and optimizing my biological networks.

Then in my midfifties I had a series of events—an infected root canal, a mold-infested house, and a broken arm—that threw my system into chaos. After taking the antibiotic for my root canal, I developed a nasty bacterial infection of my gut called C. difficile colitis as well as gastritis, where my stomach was raw and inflamed. And I was in a cytokine storm (flooded with inflammatory molecules), lost 30 pounds (13 kg), and was in bed and in and out of the hospital for five months. I was near death, according to the doctors I saw. Again, it forced me to discover new ways to heal and to reimagine medicine, to learn how to renew, rebuild, and regenerate my body from the inside out. During the COVID-19 pandemic, I had another back surgery with more complications that left me with a permanent limp and chronic pain. I learned to rebuild my physical structure through the latest advances in regenerative medicine and now am stronger than ever and pain-free. While I wish I hadn't had to go through all that suffering and pain, it taught me so much about how the body works and how to renew my health, leaving me more energetic, stronger, and healthier than I had been since my twenties.

I have incorporated many of the practices and principles I learned into the *Young Forever Program* in this book. I know the science and practice of this new medicine both as a patient and as a doctor. I have seen what may seem to be miracles: patients reversing type 2 diabetes, heart disease, high blood pressure, autoimmune diseases, depression, and even dementia, who become visibly younger using the science of functional medicine. The extraordinary ability we have to unlock the keys to disease reversal, rejuvenation, and aging backward is not a science fiction fantasy but science fact.

The principles and practices you will learn in this book will have remarkable benefits in your life. Not only will you live longer, reverse chronic disease, and shed pounds, but, more importantly, you will be filled with energy for life and work and love and play; you will be the full expression of who you came here to be. The point is not to live longer but to live better, not just to add more years to your life but to add more life to your years. While many my age are thinking about retirement and early bird specials, I am just beginning to dream about the second half of my life, the next 60 years and how I want to live. I have created a bucket list that includes wild adventures, learning new sports and languages, and living and traveling in remote and rugged places. It includes giving my knowledge, wisdom, and skills to those who need it, to contribute what I can to making this world just a little better than when I arrived, filled with a little more love and a lot more healing.

The Jewish faith has a guiding principle — *tikkun olam,* or the repair of the world, righting the wrongs, facing and addressing injustice and poverty. The gift of reaching sixty-three chronologically but being biologically decades younger gives me the energy and health to be in service of *tikkun olam.* I am on this journey as a scientist, doctor, and human who wants to explore the wonders of being alive with energy and vitality and joy. I invite you to join me on this journey, to step into a world of health and well-being beyond your wildest imagination.

So let's begin the journey, first to understand the science (I promise I will keep it simple and understandable) and then to describe the principles and practices and program that will keep you *young forever.*

Here's what you will learn:

In Part I, the *what*—the science of longevity:

- The revolution in longevity science
- How our current understanding of aging is based on abnormal aging, which is not inevitable

- How your biological age can be reversed even as you grow chronologically older
- The ten hallmarks of aging—the fundamental problems in our biology that occur with aging
- The root causes of the ten hallmarks from the perspective of functional medicine

In Part II, the *why* behind the Young Forever Program:

- How to stop and reverse biological aging: optimizing your seven core biological systems
- The science behind how to eat for longevity
- The science behind how to exercise for longevity
- The science of lifestyle practices for longevity
- How adversity and little stresses to your system (hormesis) activate longevity pathways
- The emerging advances in longevity treatments

In Part III, the *how*—the Young Forever Program:

- How to diagnose and test for the underlying causes of aging
- Using food as medicine to activate your longevity pathways
- Using nutritional supplements for enhancing health span and life span
- How to implement simple lifestyle practices and hormesis for longevity
- How to personalize your program to address your unique needs and imbalances
- My longevity routine: how I apply the longevity revolution to my own health and quest for a long and healthy life span

Let's get started!

PART I

HOW AND WHY WE AGE

Chapter 1

The Quest for the Fountain of Youth: Is Immortality Possible?

You are never too old to set another goal or to dream a new dream.

—Les Brown

Are disease and death preprogrammed events that leave us powerless victims to their inexorable approach? Or is the secret of vitality and longevity buried in our DNA, our molecules, cells, tissues, and biological networks, the interconnected ecosystem that is our human form? Longevity was common in biblical times. Methuselah died at 969 years old; Noah was 950 years old; Adam was 930 years old. Today the longest-lived fully documented human in history was the smoking, port-drinking, chocaholic Madame Jeanne Calment, a Frenchwoman who died at 122 years old. Emma Morano, an Italian woman who ate three eggs and 150 grams of raw meat a day, died at 117 years old. Circulating the internet is a video of an Arab man who claims to be 110 years old and is father to a seven-year-old son. In India I have heard personal reports of sages and rishis (Hindu saints) who live well past 150 years old. It could be that they have no birth records, or couldn't count, but that raises the question: What is the limit of human life? Is there one? If we aren't meant to have a limit, would you want to live to 150? Or beyond?

THE BLUE ZONES—LONGEVITY IN PRACTICE

There are places in the world where people have already cracked the code, without knowing it, resulting in unusual longevity. Dan Buettner, a National Geographic explorer and author, researched the places on Earth with the longest-lived, healthiest communities, called Blue Zones (after the color of the marker an earlier researcher used to circle them on a world map). These communities have up to twenty times the number of people reaching 100 years old or more than in the United States. What makes the communities unique is not their genetics—when Blue Zone inhabitants move to a more modern world, their disease and death rates parallel everyone else's. It is something else, something I have been on a quest to discover, which led me to visit the Blue Zones. What I witnessed has shaped how I view aging, longevity, and, frankly, *living*.

JOURNEYING TO SARDINIA

In the summer of 2021, with Dan's help and advice, I ventured deep into the Ogliastra region of Sardinia, the heart of Sardinia's Blue Zone, which has the longest-lived men in the world. I was guided by two native Sardinians, Eleonora Catta and Paola Demurtas, and their travel company, There, to the homes and hearths of local Sardinians, into the world of centenarians, an ancient world that has remained much the same for the last 3,000 years. The mountainous region, home to the Sardinian shepherds, is remote and landlocked and has remained inaccessible to conquerors and outside influences until recently. I heard the Sardinians' stories, witnessed their way of life, ate their ancient foods, drank their antioxidant-rich Cannonau wine.

The people of this region have preserved their ancient foodways. They still follow traditional methods of making cheese, wine, preserved meats, and olive oil and have a deep knowledge of the local plants. They understood that food was medicine even before Hippocrates! They are particular about what their goats, sheep, and pigs eat. They know that the flavors of the food come from the foods the animals eat, from the soil that feeds their plants, vegetables, and fruits. One farmer said to me, "We flavor the meat before we kill the animal." The flavor comes from phytochemicals in the plants consumed by the animals. They don't know these compounds are actually good for them. The food just tastes better. Sardinians eat some meat. They also drink goat milk, and their daily diet always includes sheep and goat cheeses.

On one side of a steep valley sat an old, abandoned, crumbling thirteenth-century village and just above it a newer one. In the 1950s the threat of a mudslide forced the villagers to evacuate and move a little farther up the mountain. At the edge of the old, abandoned village, an eighty-four-year-old shepherd, Carmine, sat on an old stone wall, his small rust-colored Panda parked next to him, driver's door open. He had pulled over when he saw us behind him and wanted to talk. Imagine that in America, someone just pulling over to the side of the road and flagging you down for a chat! He hasn't left this mountainside since 1989, when he went to visit one of his children on the Italian mainland. Carmine tends his six sheep and one goat, his chickens, and one pig amid his olive orchards, which comprise a 300-year-old olive tree among younger olive trees, growing together with pomegranates, almonds, persimmons, figs, chestnuts, and blackberries. And he grows a large garden of tomatoes, peppers, aubergines, chard, strawberries, and artichokes. He spoke of his simple life, his diet of minestrone soup, which is a staple here. Carmine's wife had died two years earlier, and he lives with his sister and her two daughters, like most Sardinians who stay in tightly knit family and friend units. His now smaller family can't eat all the food he grows, so he feeds what remains back to the animals or gives it away. His routine, the simplicity of his life, tending his animals and gardens, chatting with his friends, being useful and part of his community, and his curious mind keep him going. I asked how he spends his time when not tending his land and animals and he said he reads a lot. He opened the hatch of his Panda and pulled out a thick tome on world religions that led to a deep conversation about God, whom he is not so sure about, and climate change and the irreversible destruction of the planet. We spent three hours chatting about his life, touring his farm, and enjoying each other's company as he hiked effortlessly up and down the mountainside, calling to his sheep to come get a little ancient grain. I struggled to keep up with him as he bounded up the mountainside after his sheep.

The next day we went to visit Giulia Pisanau, who had turned 100 years old three months earlier. We talked for hours about her childhood. She was born in 1921. Her family had eleven children, and they were so poor during and after World War I they would each eat one potato a day and one egg split among all of them. She drank goat milk every day as well as minestrone soup, often with just a few courgettes and a potato. She never married and worked for a family in Cagliari, the big city in Sardinia, for decades. Then she retired and built her own home. She spent her time doing embroidery, walking around her neighborhood, and hanging out with her friends. Still sharp, she does crossword puzzles every day. Her secrets to longevity: Do not be jealous or angry, take walks, do not stress about life, and live in gratitude. She is a wealthy woman, rich in love, meaning, and purpose. And she has no ailments except a slow thyroid and a little arthritis.

The next day we visited Sylvio Bertarelli, a shepherd who lives in much the same way his ancestors have for thousands of years, on the same land perched on a mountaintop, tending his herd of 200 goats and sheep, each with its own name and personality. Sylvio and his son grow their own olives and make their own olive oil. They cultivate an ancient form of wheat called *grano cappelli* and make their own Cannonau wine, fresh goat and sheep cheeses, cured meats, and flatbreads. Sylvio lives with his wife, daughter, and son and has no Wi-Fi or computer and barely any cell service. He is surrounded by his community of twelve close childhood friends who show up for sheepshearing season and hunting excursions every year. I asked him if he experiences much stress. He paused a long while and said his biggest stress is when a goat goes missing in the middle of the night.

Everything they eat comes from their land. Tradesmen like builders are paid in cheese and milk. In the past, Sylvio and his family ate meat five times a month; now they sacrifice only the difficult animals. They eat cheese and drink milk from goats and sheep every day. During my visit, we feasted on olives, peppers, flatbread, strong cheeses, fresh goat cheese, cured meats, puffed little bread pockets (*pistoccu fritto*), pork and sheep roasted over an open wood fire, little potato-filled pasta with fresh tomato sauce (*culurgiones*), minestrone with potatoes, pasta and cour-gettes, malloreddus pasta with sausage, fresh tomatoes from the garden, and *seadas*—little fried cheese pockets drizzled with honey—for dessert, all washed down with fresh Cannonau wine served in a clay pitcher. The family runs both the farm and a restaurant, which they operate out of their house. It was an easy afternoon and evening of laughter and food and community and love.

IKARIA: A PLACE OF WILD FOOD

I visited another Blue Zone, Ikaria, Greece, and encountered much the same spirit of self-reliance, deep community, preserved ancient foodways, and an environment that naturally supports a healing diet, love and connection, and daily movement up and down the steep mountains.

Every day the Ikarians, some of the longest-lived humans on the planet, drink tea made from wild herbs, including sage. Turns out it is full of the same phytonutrients that green tea has, *epigallocatechins,* which are powerful detoxifying and anti-inflammatory antioxidants that act on our longevity switches. Is that part of the secret to their longevity? The Ikarians' diet consists mainly of wild food. Bitter and sweet wild greens. Foraged mushrooms. Wild herbal teas. All super sources of medicinal phytonutrients. The wild sage tea they drink daily has the same powerful protective longevity phytochemicals as green tea without the caffeine. They eat very little sugar—just a little preserved fruit, such as lemons and oranges, from time to time. Wild foods have the most powerful types and highest concentrations of phytonutrients, which surely contribute to their longevity. In fact, all the food is technically organic, though you'll never see a certification (or a food label at all, for that matter!). That is just how they have farmed and foraged for centuries.

I visited ninety-seven-year-old Panagiotis and his eighty-seven-year-old wife, Alkea. They were joyful, cuddly, and happy. She cooked a meal for us of wild-greens pies, fresh garden salad, and local eggs with greens and wild mushrooms served with local Ikarian wine that had not been bottled. At eighty-seven, Alkea was spry and bright-eyed, looking 20 years younger. She tended her large, terraced gardens and fruit trees and grew and preserved all their food for the year by herself, climbing the steps and steep hillside terraces with ease. Movement is built into their life. They don't retire. They wake up with more things to do than they can get done in a day, and they are surrounded by a rich community of lifelong friends and loved ones. These are the simple principles of happiness and longevity.

Younger Ikarians are preserving the old ways. Phillip, another local I visited, makes wine in the ancient ways written about by Homer. He crushes heirloom Fokiana grapes with his bare feet, pours the juice into 200-liter clay pots buried in the ground, and leaves it to ferment gently, without additives or starters. It is a fragile wine, organic only because that is how they grow the grapes, grapes that are hardened by rough soil and challenging conditions and therefore high in protective phytonutrients. He also preserved a whole leg of a pig in the traditional ways: He placed the fresh leg on a bed of grape leaves, covered it in sea salt, washed it in wine, then hung it over a fireplace and smoked it with herbs. A pig's or lamb's leg can feed his family for a whole winter. He served us steamed grape leaves and stems seasoned with sea salt and homemade olive oil, foraged wild mushrooms, fresh goat and sheep cheese, and bread made from zea flour, an ancient grain consumed by Alexander the Great to maintain his strength. Zea is also known as emmer wheat, which is high in dietary fiber, has double the protein content of regular wheat, and has far more magnesium and vitamins A, B, C, and E, while having very low levels of gluten. I left feeling happy, nourished, and loved!

It was a privilege to peek into the Sardinians' and Ikarians' ancient ways, to see the care with which they grow food and tend to their animals, the deep understanding they have that flavor originates not in the animal or plant itself but in where and how it is grown, in what the animals eat, in the wild plants rich in medicinal phytochemicals, and in the depth of the love and connection they feel toward their family, friends, and community. Science now clearly links nutrient density and the flavor of a food to its phytochemical richness—whether it is a strawberry or goat cheese or prosciutto. This is what makes food medicine; this is the type of food we want washing over our DNA, regulating our *epigenome,* the system that controls all our gene expression, and all our biological networks. These communities don't have to go to a gym, buy organic food, or mindlessly scroll through social media. Embedded in the very fabric of their lives are medicinal foods, movement up and down the mountains, deep, lifelong friendships and community, and the slow savoring of life together. We have to make adaptations in our modern lives and find good food at farmers' markets or Whole Foods, and go to the gym to work out, but there is much to learn from the Blue Zones, from the simplest practices we have drifted away from in our nuclear families and our solo, individualistic pursuits, to our removal from nature and natural cycles and knowing the source of our food. We cannot go back to live in the world of a thousand years ago, but we can learn the lessons of the Blue Zones and build our own zones within our homes, our family, our friends, and our community.

The lessons are clear. Live close to nature. Love deeply. Eat simple food raised sustainably (ideally by your own hands). Move naturally. Laugh and rest. Actually *live.* (And live longer, as it turns out.)

HEALTH SPAN VERSUS LIFE SPAN

But what does it look like to actually *live* longer? Depends on whom you ask. Most of us witness our grandparents and parents aging and getting sick, often dying long, slow, painful deaths punctuated by multiple doctor and hospital visits and supported by dozens of medications for almost as many diseases. If you're like the majority of the world witnessing the slow decline and the onslaught of chronic diseases associated with aging, living longer does not look appealing. At all. But if you ask the communities living in the Blue Zones, they'd likely tell you that living longer looks about the same as any other stage of life, just with a bit more life experience. In fact, in Dr James Fries' landmark study, "Aging, Natural Death, and the Compression of Morbidity," published in the *New England Journal of Medicine* in 1980,[1] he made it very clear that if people maintained their ideal weight, didn't smoke, and exercised regularly, they would live long, healthy, vigorous lives. And when it came time to die, they would go quickly, painlessly, and cheaply. Those who were overweight, smoked, and didn't exercise died long, painful, expensive deaths. The healthy group dramatically lengthened their years of disease-free life, that is, their health span (how long they maintained their health) and their life span (how many years they lived), while the unhealthy group often spent decades in various states of disease and dysfunction, resulting in a dramatic loss in quality of life and a burden for themselves, their families, and the health care system.

Sadly, because of our toxic diet and poor lifestyles, life expectancy in America has been on the decline since 2015, and COVID-19 has taken another three years off the life expectancy of those most burdened by chronic disease—Black, Latino, and Native American populations. The World Health Organization estimates that the average person spends the last 20 percent of their life in poor health. That's an average of about 16 years. If you live to be seventy-six years old, that means that starting at age sixty you are on your way out!

This data continues to prove that if you choose your lifestyle habits well, you can live a long, healthy life and pass quickly when the time comes.[2] In other words, your health span can equal your life span. And this is just by applying three simple lifestyle habits: don't smoke, stay at your ideal weight, and exercise. It doesn't incorporate any of the other advances we cover in *Young Forever* that will help you access a dramatically enhanced level of health and vitality.

Nobody wants to suffer. And no one wants to live to be 100 or even older in a state of disease and disability. The good news is that you won't have to if you start to incorporate the principles in this book now—whether you are ten or 100, they work! It is never too late. In fact, one *Journal of the American Medical Association* study found that starting seventy-year-old participants on a Mediterranean diet and walking regimen reduced the risk of premature death by 65 percent![3]

The prevailing view is that if people live longer, they will be a burden on society. The opposite is true if that population is healthy. They have wisdom, knowledge, and skills that can improve the social and economic well-being of society overall. And they won't cost more; in fact, extending healthy life is projected to save trillions and trillions of dollars in our economy. Dr David Sinclair, a professor of genetics at Harvard and leading aging researcher, published an analysis in *Nature Aging* entitled "The Economic Value of Targeting Aging." Through rigorous data analysis he estimated that by improving the health span of the average American (shortening or eliminating years of illness during the last 20 percent of their life) and extending life span by one year, we could save $38 trillion a year. If we extend life span across the population by 10 years, we can save $367 trillion—but only if we improve health span.[4] That is nearly ten times the total annual health care expenditure in America alone.

Today 90 percent of the United States' almost $4.1 trillion in health care expenditures is on lifestyle-preventable chronic disease—heart disease, cancer, diabetes, dementia, kidney disease, hypertension, and so on.[5] What is even more frightening is the juggernaut of disease and the overwhelm of our health care system as our currently very unhealthy population ages. A 2018 study found that 88 percent of Americans are in poor metabolic health—meaning they are on their way to heart disease and diabetes and dementia and cancer.[6] Published in 2022, just four years later, another large study found that fewer than 7 percent of Americans are metabolically healthy, in other words, have normal blood pressure, blood sugar, cholesterol, and weight, and have not had a heart attack or stroke![7] During the COVID-19 pandemic, 63 percent of hospitalizations could have been avoided by a healthy diet.[8] Those most affected by COVID are the obese, chronically ill, and elderly (who nearly all have a chronic disease).

The moral of the story: Focusing on staying healthy pays big dividends in both the quality and length of our lives as we age, and it is never too late to start.

Health Span versus Life Span

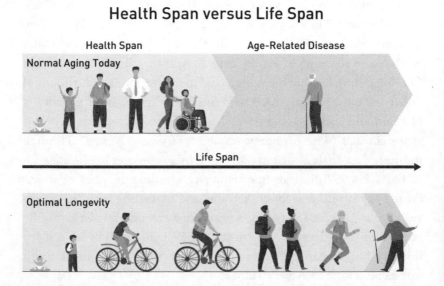

Most of the villagers I met in the Blue Zones have a health span equal to their life span. Many arrive at 100 years old active, healthy, imbued with a sense of purpose, and connected in a deep web of community. Obviously, the goal is not to become a shepherd or live in a mountain village. The key is to integrate the habits and behaviors that consistently have been proven to prevent disease and enhance your vitality and quality of life. Each of us would achieve the same longevity, filled with vibrant health, joy, and fulfillment. How do we do that? You don't have to ditch your phone, your job, or your home, or change your genes. By following the principles and the plan in *Young*

Forever you can look forward to a longer life, a life where your health span equals your life span.

LONGEVITY SCIENCE: REIMAGINING AGING

Before you dismiss the idea that biological aging is an inevitable part of life, imagine if we considered aging a disease. Like other diseases it would have a cause, symptoms, and a natural history. If we didn't address this disease, eventually we'd die, just as we would from other diseases. Imagine if we reframed our approach to aging. To do this, we must challenge a few entrenched beliefs about aging.

First: We must imagine that getting older doesn't inevitably mean getting weaker, slower, sicker, feebler, or more dependent. Almost everyone knows someone in their nineties who still dances, cooks, drives, spends time with loved ones, reads books, does puzzles, and thoroughly enjoys being alive. It shouldn't be an anomaly but the norm. Hiking, skydiving, living, and loving past 100 years old should be what we expect.

Second: We must disrupt the existing medical paradigm. The practice of medicine today is reductionist and siloed and ignores the current science that has revealed the body to be one whole integrated system or network. If you have psoriasis, arthritis, heart disease, diabetes, irritable bowel, and depression you may be referred to six different specialists, but all these problems are caused by inflammation. You will be given the best drugs to treat the symptoms of each disease based on the latest medical research, but none of the specialists is likely to address the disease's root cause. For example, food sensitivities as well as imbalances in the gut and microbiome can cause all these conditions and diseases. They are not separate and distinct problems. Treat the cause or causes, and the symptoms and diseases disappear.

Your body is not a set of independent organs. It is a weblike ecosystem. The same root cause can result in multiple different symptoms and conditions. Address the causes and provide the conditions for health, and diseases go away as a side effect.

FUNCTIONAL MEDICINE: A NEW APPROACH TO HEALTH CARE

In the groundbreaking textbook from Harvard scientists called *Network Medicine: Complex Systems in Disease and Therapeutics,* the authors present a radically different view of medicine, a model that challenges our current organ-based, single-disease, single-drug model. They explain it this way: "Network medicine embraces the complexity of multifactorial influences on disease. While network medicine offers a fundamentally different approach toward understanding disease etiology (cause), it will eventually lead to key differences in how diseases are treated—with multiple molecular targets that may require manipulation in a coordinated, dynamic fashion."

The authors referred to this radically different approach to health care as "network medicine"; I and many of my colleagues call it "functional medicine." Functional medicine suggests that all diseases have a root cause (etiology). We must find and address all the factors or causes that contribute to disease. If your roof is leaking, you need to find the hole and patch it. And if you have multiple holes, you must fix them all. The good news is that most of the root causes are treatable through diet and lifestyle interventions—practices available to almost anyone. This approach will change how we treat disease. Rather than suppressing symptoms with medication, we can map out the root causes and address all of them with multiple simultaneous interventions that restore and enhance optimal function. *Functional medicine is the science of creating health.* When you create health, disease disappears.

The body comprises seven dynamically interconnected, networked systems that underlie all disease—155,000 diseases, in fact. What are these systems?

1. Assimilating nutrients, digestion, and the microbiome
2. Defense and repair (immune and inflammatory system)
3. Energy production (mitochondria)
4. Detoxification

5. Transportation (circulation and lymphatic system)
6. Communication (hormones, neurotransmitters, etc.)
7. The body's structure (from cellular structures to the musculo-skeletal system)

When these systems are in dynamic balance, health and longevity are the natural consequences. Disrupt any system and disease and aging occur. Functional medicine provides a road map to assess all the environmental, lifestyle, and predisposing factors—genes, stress, toxins, trauma, microbes, diet, allergens, and so on, that cause imbalance in these systems. We identify the *what* (symptoms) and the *why* (too much or too little of what is needed for health) so we can determine the *how* (removing the impediments to health and adding the ingredients for health). This allows us to focus on the personalized strategies for lifestyle interventions and managing our environment to create the best outcomes, prevent chronic disease, and extend healthy life span.

Functional medicine asks a different series of questions than traditional medicine does. How do we create health? How do we optimize function? How do we reverse dysfunction caused by the normal ravages of our modern world where most of us live and eat in a toxic food and nutritional wasteland, where we sit most of the day, where we live in a sea of toxic industrial chemicals, where the stress of our lives and society and global existential threats like climate change and totalitarianism and the digital persuasion economy that drives our thoughts, emotions, and actions are usurping our free will?

Within our bodies is a powerful innate healing system. We simply need to activate it by removing and avoiding the inputs that negatively impact our seven systems and provide what these systems need to function optimally. Put simply: take out the bad stuff, put in the good stuff. The Young Forever Program is designed to do just that, and to activate our innate healing system to prevent and reverse disease and help you live longer and better.

THE FUTURE OF MEDICINE IS HERE

This book is a road map to extending both your health span and your life span using the science and tools available today. Emerging advances in technology and longevity science are pushing the limits of our imagination, but even without the promise of these advances we can take advantage of revolutionary discoveries in the field of longevity. We now know how to control our master longevity switches through diet, lifestyle, supplements, and even medication and arrive at 100 years old in good health. We can reverse disease, enhance our bodies' repair systems, regenerate and repair cells and tissues, and turn back our biological clock. Getting to 120 or 150 or 200 (while still feeling youthful and vibrant) will soon be possible with therapies and innovations just on the horizon. If you can maintain your health for another 10 or 15 years you will be alive when we might reach *longevity escape velocity*— when our scientific advances will keep pushing death off indefinitely.

In laboratories and research centers around the world, research on aging is accelerating exponentially. Massive private investment in aging research is driving these innovations. The world's billionaires are doubling down on funding this research—Google's biotech company Calico, Jeff Bezos and Yuri Milner's investment in Altos Labs, XPRIZE, and others are pouring billions into aging research, dwarfing the research budget of the National Institutes of Health. We are also in an exponential phase of scientific progress and discovery made possible by innovations in systems biology, artificial intelligence, nanotechnology, quantum computing, and more. Leading aging researchers suggest we will reach longevity escape velocity in 15 years.[9] However, George Church, professor of genetics at Harvard and MIT, suggests we may already be there. In his lab, reversal of age-related biomarkers and pathologies has already been achieved in human cells and animal aging models. It's hard to imagine, but real healthy life extension just may be possible soon.[10] Our minds think in linear, not exponential terms. Thirty linear steps will get you about 30 meters. Thirty exponential steps will take you twenty-six times around the

Earth. If I gave you $1 a day for thirty days, you would have $30. If I gave you 1 cent but doubled it every day, in thirty days you would have $10 million. Our minds struggle to comprehend the power of exponential change.

Consider for a moment the startling recent discovery of *Yamanaka factors* (known formally as Oct3/4, Sox2, Klf4, c-Myc). Shinya Yamanaka won the Nobel Prize for his discovery that these factors control which genes in a cell are turned on or off, ensuring that embryonic cells differentiate into the cells they were meant to become. A brain cell knows to be a brain cell. A skin cell becomes a skin cell. Yamanaka proved that, using these factors, we could create iPSCs — *induced pluripotent stem cells,* which can become any cell in the body.[11] This means that you can reprogram your genes to create a younger you. These factors can take any cell back to its undifferentiated youthful, newborn state. We can now do this in animals. Imagine scraping off a few skin cells, and, like Benjamin Button, reverse engineering them to become essentially embryonic cells that could become a new pancreas or heart or brain. Soon we will be able to take your own stem cells and make them even younger than young — embryonic — and turn them into any cell in the body that needs repair. Hip and knee replacements and heart and kidney transplants will become the stuff of history books, an archaic treatment akin to bloodletting.

Much research is still needed to safely apply this technique in humans, but in animal models Yamanaka factors are reversing aging and repairing organs. This is just one discovery in hundreds that are pulling back the veil on the causes of aging and the science of how to reverse aging, to reprogram, regenerate, rejuvenate, and repair your body. It is not one thing we need to do but many. It is not one cause but many that drive the dysfunction we see as aging and disease. And the good news is we are closer than ever to understanding how it all works.

Many species defy the limits of what we imagine as a normal life span. Greenland sharks live up to 400 years, bowhead whales may live over 200 years, and Galapagos tortoises live over 150 years; some scientists think tortoises may live up to 400 or 500 years. Scientists working at the frontiers of aging can consistently extend life in animals by 30 percent or more, equivalent to humans reaching 120 years old. In some yeast models they can extend life to the equivalent of 1,000 years.

The alchemists of yore sought the fountain of youth in gold and special potions. They were the longevity scientists of their day. However, today we are perched on the edge of a radical reconceptualization of health and disease unlike anything before in medicine. Imagine living in the 1500s, before the discovery of the microscope, before Antoni van Leeuwenhoek discovered bacteria in 1676, before Louis Pasteur proposed the germ theory of disease—an infection might be viewed as a visitation by evil spirits or an imbalance in the humors or the hex of a witch. Those discoveries heralded a new era in medicine. Today we are on the edge of an even greater paradigm shift about disease and aging.

Powerful advances in technology, computing, and medicine are about to flip our whole model of diagnosis and treatment on its head. Diagnosing diseases today is like listening to the noises a car makes and trying to figure out what's wrong rather than looking under the hood. We are profoundly good at naming all the noises (i.e., diseases) based on the symptoms they produce but have very little understanding of the *why*. The new medicine will allow us to look under the hood, hook up the car's computer to a supercomputer, then map out every disturbance, learn what needs fixing, and fix it.

All this may seem like science fiction, but it is closer to reality than most of us imagine. The good news is that the foundational tenets of healthy aging do not need more proof. The steps needed to prevent, reverse, and even cure most of the chronic diseases that drive rapid aging and death are already proven, and available to almost everyone—what we eat, how we move, rest, and sleep, how socially connected we are, and more.

In *Young Forever,* we'll explore our current understanding of the underlying biology of aging—not just diseases but the *hallmarks of aging,* the things that seem to go universally wrong as we age, and that underlie all the diseases of aging. If we treat the hallmarks and their causes, then we don't need to treat heart disease or cancer or diabetes or dementia.

The scientific advances around the hallmarks of aging are being informed by the recognition that our biology is an information system, a network of networks, dynamically balancing all our biological functions, managing and coordinating literally trillions and trillions of molecular events every second. Functional medicine goes one step further and addresses the *root causes of the hallmarks of aging*. For example, one of the hallmarks is inflammation. But rather than treat inflammation with new or better medication (i.e., anti-inflammatories or NSAIDs), functional medicine addresses the root causes of inflammation—toxins, allergens, microbiome imbalances, infections, stress, and poor diet, as well as a lack of the ingredients needed to create health, including whole real food, nutrients, the right balance of hormones, light, clean water and air, movement, rest, sleep, love, community, meaning, and purpose. Address the root causes and inflammation goes away.

We can improve our health span *and* our life span by combining advances in technology with the road map of functional medicine. Some of these advances are changing everything we know about the practice of medicine. They include:

- Functional medicine
- The omics revolution—the mapping of the human genome, transcriptome, proteome, metabolome, microbiome, sociogenome, and so on
- Quantified-self measurement tools, including Function Health whole body lab testing, the Oura Ring, Levels Health continuous glucose monitoring, the Whoop, Apple Watch, Eight Sleep, and, soon, more advanced implantable biosensors that measure your biochemistry in real time
- Advances in artificial intelligence and machine learning that will analyze billions of personal data points, identify patterns and

imbalances, and help create a personalized map for enhancing every aspect of your biology

- Quantum computing, which can process enormous amounts of biological information

Even before these trends become everyday realities in the practice of medicine (which is often decades behind the advances in science), simple, proven dietary, lifestyle, behavioral, and environmental changes available today can radically transform our health.

The story of Katherine, a patient at our Center for Functional Medicine at Cleveland Clinic, will make you stop and think about what is possible. Katherine was sixty-six when she came to see us, severely obese, suffering from clogged arteries that needed stents, heart failure, high blood pressure, fatty liver, failing kidneys, and type 2 diabetes on insulin. Her blood tests were scary, and she was on her way to a heart and kidney transplant. She was on a pile of medications for which her co-pay was $20,000 (£17,000) a year. Within three days of joining our group program, by changing her diet from a lifetime of junk food to using food as medicine, consuming a very low-glycemic, high-fiber, good-fat, phytonutrient-rich, plant-rich diet, and following a simple vitamin regimen (multivitamin, fish oil, and vitamin D) she was able to get off her insulin. Within three months she was off all her medication and her numbers were all normal (heart failure gone, kidneys and liver normalized, and blood pressure and blood sugar normal). After a year she lost 116 pounds (52 kg) and was able to fully return to a vibrant, active life as a leader in her community.

No dieting, no organ transplants.

By not even taking advantage of the radical discoveries in longevity science, just applying the simple principles of functional medicine, Katherine's body was able to repair, renew, and regenerate after six decades of abuse and neglect. The body has within it instructions for repair. We simply must provide the right conditions to activate the body's innate healing systems.

And with the new discoveries in the field of aging and the science of rejuvenation, we will be able to go beyond just reversing disease; we will be able to restore your molecules and cells and tissues to a younger state. *Young Forever* provides the foundational principles that you can apply now and incorporates today's leading discoveries that may safely extend life. And what's around the corner has the potential to dramatically improve the quality and length of life beyond our wildest imagination. We will cover that too!

Chapter 2

The Root Causes of Aging

I want to know how God created this world. I am not interested in this or that phenomenon, in the spectrum of this or that element; I want to know his thoughts; the rest are details.

—ALBERT EINSTEIN

If I asked you what the biggest risk factor for death was, you might say heart disease or cancer—the two diseases that seem to kill the most people. However, if we completely eradicated both heart disease and cancer from the planet, the human life span would increase only five to seven years, far from the goal of getting to age 100 or 120 (but only in good health). You might say smoking and obesity are the biggest causes of chronic disease and death, and you would be partially right. But if you look at a thirty-year-old smoker versus a seventy-year-old nonsmoker, who has a greater risk of cancer, heart attacks, and death? Smoking may increase your risk of cancer fivefold. Aging increases it fifty-fold.

More than anything else, aging itself accelerates the risk of chronic disease. Why?

Aging is a disease.

What do we see as the "average" person ages in the Western world? Most of us imagine aging as a loss of function and ability, a time of illness, medications, and doctors' visits. Those kinds of issues may be your biggest concerns, a nagging worry about your health span. Even if you eat real, whole foods and exercise regularly, you've probably noticed changes that come with age that you just can't seem to control—fatigue, lower energy, poorer fitness levels, poor sleep, aches and pains, lower sex drive, loss of muscle, worsening vision and hearing, digestive problems, memory loss. Those are the early warning signs of aging as a disease in itself. They are *not* inevitable consequences of getting *chronologically* older, but they are signs of getting *biologically* older.

Every system in our body is affected by *biological aging:* our microbiome, our immune system, hormones, metabolism and energy production, detoxification systems, circulatory and lymph systems, and our structural system. We see progressive neuropsychological changes, including a global decline in neurotransmitter production, declining ability to respond to stress, slowed cognitive processing, impaired memory, lowered pain threshold and chronic pain, and decreasing sensory acuity in sight, hearing, and balance. We also see changes in our musculoskeletal system, including loss of flexibility, loss of muscle, loss of cardiovascular fitness, and degenerative joint disease (also known as osteoarthritis).

We lose significant amounts of muscle, resulting in *sarcopenia* (literally, "less muscle") and weakness and frailty. Our energy decreases. Our adrenal glands have trouble keeping up with the stresses of life. And our energy factories, or mitochondria, degrade and slow down. What's the difference between a three-year-old who runs around with boundless energy and a ninety-year-old who moves very slowly? The number and function of their mitochondria. We become more insulin resistant and pre-diabetic and have trouble regulating our blood sugar; our blood vessels stiffen, causing high blood pressure; our weight typically increases as our fat mass goes up and our muscle mass goes down; and we gain weight more easily because muscle burns seven times the calories of fat.

We become more nutrient deficient. We lose our appetite, and our ability to absorb nutrients decreases. Our immune system declines in function, so we are more susceptible to flu and pneumonia and other infections. This is why COVID-19 disproportionately kills the elderly. In fact, our immune system struggles to fight infection and cancer and heal wounds. But low-grade systemic inflammation increases, accelerating all the diseases of aging. And while our immune system is underactive in fighting outside invaders, it becomes more susceptible to autoimmunity, where the immune system turns against itself. Our microbiome degrades, resulting in leaky gut and even more inflammation. All in all, not a pretty picture. These all lead to what may seem like an inevitable outcome: the diseases of aging.

Following are the diseases that burden most people as they age. They cause early disability, decline in function, and premature death.

- Pre-diabetes and type 2 diabetes
- Cardiovascular disease (heart attack, stroke, heart failure, and high blood pressure)
- Cancer
- Cognitive decline and dementia
- Renal failure
- Hormonal imbalances (thyroid, adrenal, sex hormones, growth hormone)
- Sarcopenia (muscle loss)
- Osteoporosis (bone loss)
- Autoimmunity
- Macular degeneration and cataracts
- Lung disease (mostly from smoking)

According to the CDC, six in ten Americans have one of the conditions noted above and four in ten have two or more. More than 80 percent of people over sixty-five have one or more of these problems.[1] No wonder they seem to be a "normal" part of aging. But they are not. They are signs of abnormal aging, of accelerated damage and dysfunction resulting in the *hallmarks of aging*. We will see how treating the root causes of aging can address all these diseases (and the consequences in Chapter 4) without treating the disease directly. And for those who have more end-stage versions of aging-related diseases, emerging innovations in science will help to create new organs, reprogram your cells to a younger you, and heal and repair damaged cells and tissues. Some of these are on the near horizon, some farther off, but what we know now can have a powerful impact on your health and literally reverse your biological age.

WHAT CREATES THE DISEASE OF AGING?

The diseases listed in the previous section cause prolonged suffering, disability, and death. The average eighty-year-old has five diseases and takes five medications. It sounds dismal, but by reframing how we approach aging and treating it like a disease, we can reimagine a healthier, longer life, a life where we can prevent, treat, and even reverse these seemingly inevitable consequences of getting older. We spend billions on disease research, but mostly on the wrong things. *Aging* results in 85 percent of health care costs and yet accounts for only 6 percent of government research spending (and most of that is spent on the diseases of aging rather than on the biology of aging itself).

If we do not take care of ourselves, if we do not activate our healing programs and longevity switches, if we go about our business as usual, the diseases of aging will take hold and degrade our bodies over time. Decay and disintegration and disorganization are facts of life. The laws of physics subject all systems to entropy (breakdown). However, if we provide our bodies with the right information, energy, and inputs, we can stop and reverse the entropy of aging. In fact, our bodies are designed both to clean up and repair old cells and proteins and to build new molecules, cells, and tissues. Both these functions are needed for life. The problem with aging is imbalance: too much decay and not enough rebuilding. Just as an old car or old house needs extra care to stay functional, so do we. Unfortunately, our modern diet and lifestyle primarily drive the slow decay of our biology. We do not take

advantage of the diet and lifestyle habits and other innovative strategies available today to activate the healing, repair, and regeneration
process that is embedded in our DNA.

Yes, we can better "manage" these diseases today than we could
100 years ago. But I don't want you to have to manage them. I want to
prevent them entirely and reverse them completely. That might seem
fantastical, but as you will learn, scientific advances in understanding
the biology of aging and disease are forcing us to radically reconsider
our approach from whack-a-mole medicine, treating each disease separately, to reimagining health and disease as signs of dysfunction with
root causes that can be modified and treated to create health.

Scientists have mapped the ways in which things go wrong as we
get chronologically older. They have identified ten hallmarks of aging,
changes in our biology that are upstream to the diseases they cause:

1. Disrupted hormone and nutrient signaling—food and aging
2. DNA damage and mutations—problems with our genetic
    blueprint
3. Telomere shortening—becoming unraveled
4. Damaged proteins—malformed, misshapen, dysfunctional
    molecules
5. Epigenetic damage—a dysfunctional piano player
6. Senescent cells—the attack of the zombies
7. Depleted energy—the decline of our mitochondria
8. Of microbes and men—the link between gut health and
    longevity
9. Stem cell exhaustion—the decline of our body's rejuvenation
    system
10. Inflammaging—the fire that drives chronic disease and short-
    ens life

We will cover these hallmarks in detail in Chapter 4. The good news
is that we know how to address problems with the hallmarks with simple
lifestyle and behavior changes and the science of functional medicine. It

is as simple as this: out with the bad, in with the good. We must remove and avoid the things that harm our health, including poor diet, stress, sedentary lifestyle, toxins, allergens, and microbes (the bad stuff); and add in the ingredients for health, including whole real food, nutrients, the right balance of hormones, clean water and air, light, sleep, movement, rest, community, love, meaning, and purpose (the good stuff).

It sounds simple, and the good news is that it is. When we avoid and remove the negative inputs that harm our biology and drive disease and add in the healing factors, nutrients, and things that allow our bodies to function optimally, we can heal and reverse abnormal aging. Before we get to that, let's take a deeper look at the failure of our current approach to the diseases of aging.

THE DISEASES OF AGING: ARE THEY ALL JUST ONE DISEASE?

Medicine today makes a diagnosis by assessing symptoms and physical signs and sometimes running a few lab tests and imaging studies. We have become very good at describing diseases according to symptoms but not at addressing the root causes of disease. Our current model can work well especially for acute care, like a broken bone or a heart attack. Thank God for emergency medicine and surgery. But for chronic lifestyle diseases of aging it doesn't work as well.

The current health care model (truthfully a *sick care* model) focuses on naming diseases and suppressing symptoms. Some cures are possible with surgery and some with medication, but they are the exceptions. That is why 80 percent of what ails Americans and increasingly the global population is "chronic" disease — disease that requires long-term management but is rarely cured. From migraines to multiple sclerosis, from diabetes to dementia, from asthma to autism, from cancer to colitis. Why is it that we are advancing science and technology so rapidly in medicine and yet all chronic illness is on the rise, creating devastation for families, societies, economies, and nations? Doing more of the same will not solve our chronic disease problem, nor will it provide a road map to creating optimal health and longevity.

If you have pain in your head, you are likely to receive a diagnosis of a "headache," but this could be a symptom of many different things. Giving pain medication might help the headache but won't address the root cause or causes. There are many things that can hurt your head, but only so many ways it can say "ouch." It could be you have a migraine, or a brain tumor, or an aneurysm, or are allergic to gluten, or are just stressed-out or dehydrated. Without understanding what causes the pain in the first place, you'll end up with a lifetime of pain, medication, frustration, doctors' bills, and both a figurative and literal headache. Treating symptoms is currently how we approach most diseases like cancer, heart disease, dementia, diabetes, autoimmune disease, and more. But we are not making headway, as the incidence of these diseases continues to rise. Doing more of the same won't fix the problem.

For example, more than $2 billion (£1.6 billion) has been spent on more than 400 studies aiming to treat and cure Alzheimer's, and not a single truly useful medication has been discovered (at best, a few showed delayed admission to a nursing home by a few months). What about the *why*? *Why* does Alzheimer's exist? What is the *cause*? Preventing this disease in the first place, and even reversing it by identifying and understanding the root causes, is far more important than merely delaying the onset of symptoms by a few months.

For the last 30 years functional medicine has incorporated the advances in systems biology and network medicine into a practical clinical model to reverse disease and create optimal health. It has been mostly on the margins of medicine, but in 2014 the legendary CEO of Cleveland Clinic, Toby Cosgrove, invited me to start the Cleveland Clinic Center for Functional Medicine to bring this paradigm to the forefront of health care. Functional medicine is a way of connecting the dots, an approach that has taken the underlying science of the body's systems and networks and turned it into a practical, scalable clinical model for assessing disturbances in the systems that give rise to disease, and for optimizing those networks to create health and longevity.

Functional medicine forces us to reimagine disease and treatment. Most diseases of aging result from the same underlying correctable *imbalances*. Too much or too little of the things that drive imbalances in our body's seven physiological systems drive the hallmarks of aging and the diseases that result from those fixable dysfunctions.

For example, what do Alzheimer's, heart disease, cancer, diabetes, obesity, and even some cases of infertility and depression have in common? All can result from an imbalance in blood sugar and insulin resistance. This problem is, as we will see, at the root of much of the aging process. It now affects more than nine in ten Americans and is the result of our highly processed high-sugar and high-starch diet and sedentary lifestyle. Doctors miss up to 90 percent of cases. *It's also nearly 100 percent reversible.*

What causes insulin resistance? Too much starch and sugar! Described simply, when you eat anything that breaks down into sugar—like bread, pastas, crackers, desserts, sugar-sweetened beverages, and starches like rice and potatoes—your pancreas releases insulin, a hormone that's responsible for taking the sugar (glucose) from your bloodstream and delivering it to your cells for energy. The more starch and sugar you eat, the more insulin you produce in order to clear the sugars from your bloodstream. Insulin is the *fat-storage hormone*. Over time, your cells become resistant to the effects of insulin, requiring more and more to keep your blood sugar normal. Higher insulin results in a cascade of harmful effects. Storage of dangerous belly fat, loss of muscle, increased hunger and sugar cravings, inflammation, high blood pressure, worsening cholesterol profile (low HDL, high triglycerides, small LDL particles), fatty liver, altered sex hormones and sexual dysfunction, depression, memory loss, increased blood clotting, and ultimately type 2 diabetes, heart attacks, strokes, dementia, and cancer. Treating all these conditions separately with medication becomes unnecessary when we reverse insulin resistance, when we address the root cause. These are not separate problems. They are more like branches on a tree with the same roots and trunk. Functional medicine addresses the soil and roots, not the branches and leaves (symptoms and diseases). In fact, I almost never treat disease; I create health in my patients and the diseases just disappear.

FUNCTIONAL MEDICINE AND THE INFORMATION THEORY OF AGING

The science of living *better and longer* is already here . . . if we focus on *why* diseases of aging occur, the root causes. We don't treat diseases through functional medicine; we treat the system, not the symptoms. The future of medicine and longevity treatments must focus on treating the whole system. To do that, we need to understand systems biology and the *information theory of aging,* a framework first proposed by Dr David Sinclair.

Max Planck famously said, "A new scientific truth does not triumph by convincing its opponents and making them see the light, but rather because its opponents eventually die, and a new generation grows up that is familiar with it." In other words, medicine advances one funeral at a time. I wish we could move faster than that, but breaking through the paradigm of "normal" science is extraordinarily difficult, whether overturning the belief that the Earth is flat or that the sun revolves around the Earth or that species evolve through natural selection (still being debated more than 160 years later). Functional medicine, the science of approaching our biology as a whole and understanding that our seven core biological systems (discussed in Chapter 6) are intimately interconnected, is a profound paradigm shift in our understanding of health and disease. It turns medicine upside down. The entire system of medical education and practice and our health insurance system are based on outdated notions of disease. Our current systems are based on describing diseases according to symptoms, not on diagnosing and treating root causes (such as diet, lifestyle, or environmental factors). It is a difficult ship to turn, but turning it is imperative if we are to halt the juggernaut of chronic disease advancing despite the best efforts of our well-meaning (but outdated) health care system. Ignoring and delaying the adoption of this scientific revolution in medical practice will result in millions suffering and dying needlessly. Applying systems thinking to the disease of aging has the potential to radically shift health care, making the future of medicine available today.

Functional medicine can keep your body running in an optimal disease-free, high-performance state for decades and decades. The information theory of aging suggests that disease occurs because of corrupted information in our biological networks, like damaged software code that results in altered signals that prevent our innate healing and repair systems from doing their job. Functional medicine addresses the causes and repairs the corrupted software code.

Scientists have discovered how to activate the body's own healing and repair mechanisms, turning on the right genes, activating the right molecules, and providing the body with the right inputs to rebuild and renew our bodies. Think of a house remodel. First you need to get rid of old parts and structures—the demo and recycling phase. Next comes the rebuild and construction needed to create the new home. The same is true for the human body. We have a built-in demo, cleanup, and recycling system as well as a renewal and construction system. Our modern lifestyle and habits and environment all push us into disease, impeding both the demo and construction systems built into our biology. Functional medicine provides the blueprint to optimize both breakdown of old parts and renewal of our biological systems, allowing us to stay healthy and functional even as centenarians.

Medical specialization will become obsolete as we now understand that all the diseases of aging have the same roots, and by treating the roots we can prevent, treat, and likely reverse course. In a very real sense, all the diseases of aging are a single disease (imbalance) located in slightly different places in the body and manifesting in slightly different ways, depending on your genetic and environmental predispositions. If we address all the underlying hallmarks, we don't need to treat each disease separately. We treat the root causes, the imbalances, and all the downstream diseases go away.

This century is witness to the most dramatic changes in our

understanding of biology in the last 150 years. Not since the discovery of evolution or cells or bacteria has there been such a radical reimagining of biology. It echoes the shift from Newtonian to quantum physics. It is changing everything we know about how to diagnose and treat disease, and how to create health and longevity.

The basic work of science is to break things down into parts, into the smallest fragments of knowledge. But science must be paired with synthesis, zooming out to see how the pieces fit and work together. Your body didn't go to medical school. It didn't get the memo that it is supposed to organize itself into medical specialties. It is one whole ecosystem. Every second there are trillions and trillions of chemical reactions happening at the speed of light inside you. It is like a symphony with millions of instruments that must all play in coordination to make music. *Young Forever* will help you become the conductor of this beautiful symphony.

A CASE STUDY IN FUNCTIONAL MEDICINE: TREATING THE SYSTEM, NOT THE SYMPTOMS

Scientists at the leading edge of longevity research have mapped out the changes in our biology associated with aging, the hallmarks of aging. This is a huge step forward in looking under the hood to see what's wrong, what systems degrade or malfunction as we age. They are deep into studying how to treat and reverse these hallmarks of aging in the hope that we can prolong life and stop chronic disease. These scientists talk not about treating or curing different age-related diseases but about going upstream to get to the root mechanisms that underlie all diseases.

This is the medicine I have practiced for 30 years with remarkable patient outcomes. I am often witness to miracles. Except they are not miracles, just the expected result from applying this theory of medicine to real people.

Let me give you an example. A forty-nine-year-old female executive business coach came to see me at Cleveland Clinic with a whole list of problems (that's why I call myself a holistic doctor, because I treat people with a "whole list" of problems). She had a severe autoimmune disease called psoriatic arthritis, which was treated with a powerful immuno-suppressive medication that cost $50,000 (£42,000) a year. She was also depressed, overweight, and pre-diabetic and suffered from migraines, irritable bowel syndrome, and reflux. After seeing the best specialists for each disease, she was put on the best current treatments, what we call the standard of care. The psychiatrist put her on an antidepressant, the endocrinologist prescribed metformin for her blood sugar, and the gas-troenterologist gave her acid blockers and antispasmodic medication for her gut. Lastly her neurologist gave her the best migraine treatment medication. And while some of her symptoms were "managed"—in other words, minimized—they were not gone and neither were her diseases. In short, she was miserable and desperate.

I asked a different set of questions. How are all those conditions connected? Inflammation. Yes, even depression is inflammation of the brain. But rather than give her drugs to shut off the inflammation, I asked a simple question. Why was her immune system so angry? Where were the imbalances?

I quickly figured out that the source of most of her diseases was her gut. Seventy percent of the immune system is in the gut, and it was clear her microbiome was out of balance.[2] She had been on lots of ste-roids and antibiotics, which promote the growth of bad bugs and kill the good ones. When she ate, she would get a "bloated stomach," or severe bloating, suggesting overgrowth of bad bacteria and yeast in her gut. This was a clue she had leaky gut; the barrier keeping poop and undigested food particles inside the intestinal tract was damaged, causing a flood of foreign molecules into her bloodstream activating her immune system. She was also likely low in healthy gut bacteria and low in vitamin D.

All I did was reset and balance her gut. I took out the inflamma-tory processed foods and dairy and gluten (often big triggers for inflammation). And I gave her an antibiotic that doesn't get absorbed into the bloodstream to kill off the bad bugs causing her bloated stomach and an antifungal for all the yeast in her system from antibiotics and steroids. In other words, we took out the bad stuff.

Then I added in good stuff using food as medicine—nutrient-dense, low-glycemic, anti-inflammatory foods along with probiotics, fish oil, vitamin D, and a multivitamin.

I didn't treat her diseases; I simply rebooted and restored her gut ecosystem, which was at the root of all her diseases and symptoms. Six weeks later she came back and reported that not only were her psoriasis and arthritis gone but she had no more migraines, depression, reflux, or irritable bowel, and she had lost 20 pounds (9 kg) and reversed her pre-diabetes. And despite my instructions to stay on her medication, she stopped everything and was better than ever. This case is not an anomaly but a routine outcome from applying functional medicine.

As a functional medicine doctor, my job is to be a medical detective, to root out the impediments to and add in the ingredients for health and longevity. Working to solve the root causes of accelerated aging and disease must be the first step. Even without any more advances in the science of aging, we are missing the low-hanging fruit, simple practices that can extend life at least 10 or 20 more years. Then we can use all the emerging tools and technologies to repair damage that has been done and to activate longevity switches and pathways that go beyond just good health, that launch us into a revolutionary new epoch in medicine that may help us reach 120 years old in good health and maybe even reach longevity escape velocity.

Chapter 3

Biological versus Chronological Age

We don't stop playing because we grow old. We grow old because we stop playing.

— George Bernard Shaw

I am sixty-three, born in 1959. There is no changing that. Unless I go far out into space for a long time and return much younger than those I left behind (thanks to Einstein's laws of relativity), I can't change my chronological age. But what about my biological age? Your birthday determines your chronological age, but what determines the age of your biology? It turns out that though they are often related and track in time, your biological age can accelerate or reverse at any point in time based on the inputs to your biology. Recent advances in science allow us to measure your biological age.

At the very end of each of your chromosomes is a telomere, a protective little cap, like the plastic tip at the end of your shoelaces that prevents them from unraveling. Telomeres shorten as we age and eventually can't hold the shoelaces, the DNA double helix, from unraveling, and then we die. Elizabeth Blackburn won a Nobel Prize for her discovery of *telomerase,* the enzyme that helps lengthen telomeres. She also discovered that telomerase activity increases through a healthy diet and lifestyle, lengthening telomeres and your life. Your telomeres provide a running real-time snapshot of how you are biologically aging. You can test your telomeres through a simple saliva or blood test at commercial labs. At fifty-eight years old, I tested mine, and the biological age of my telomeres was thirty-nine years old, almost 20 years younger than my chronological age.

A better method to measure biological age was recently developed by Steve Horvath, a human geneticist and biostatistician at the University of California, Los Angeles.[1] Having a way to measure biological age is essential because without valid ways to measure the effects of any lifestyle or pharmaceutical intervention on our true rate of aging, it would be difficult to draw meaningful conclusions about what works or doesn't to reverse biological aging. Dr Horvath has discovered a way to measure biological age by measuring the *epigenetic clock,* also known as the Horvath clock, which reflects how your gene expression changes and interacts with your environment throughout your life. Your lifestyle and environment alter your gene expression. By measuring something called *DNA methylation,* the chemical tags or bookmarks on your genes that determine which genes are read (turned on) or silenced (turned off), you can determine your biological age. Studies have shown that a few simple functional medicine dietary and lifestyle interventions can reverse biological age (measured by DNA methylation) by three years in just two short months.[2] Measuring DNA methylation is available to all of us now, and I encourage you to use it to measure the effects of the Young Forever Program over time (see Part III).

EPIGENETICS: THE MASTER REGULATOR OF HEALTH AND LONGEVITY

The key to understanding our biological age requires a short primer on genetics: DNA, *epigenetics,* and a very important biochemical process happening billions of times a second in your body called *methylation.* Take a ride with me into understanding this critical process that determines nearly everything about our health and longevity.

Let's start at the beginning.

Your DNA, also known as your genome. Each of us has a unique genetic code inherited from our parents. Think of your DNA as computer hardware that controls your biological functions. A computer uses a binary code of ones and zeros. Whether you're typing on a laptop word processor or creating a full-blown *Matrix*-like virtual reality, it all results from a combination of ones and zeros. Your DNA is exponentially more complex and powerful than computer coding. Your book of life is written with four compounds called *nucleotides,* represented by the letters A (adenine), G (guanine), C (cytosine), and T (thymine). The average human has 6 billion of these nucleotides with combinations of AGCT that are unique to you. Each gene is comprised of three of these nucleotides linked together in a specific order, such as ACT or GTA. You have about 20,000 genes, much the same as an earthworm. What makes you different from an earthworm are slight variations in the code, spelling changes such as swapping a T for a C that change the function of the proteins produced from that gene. Humans have between 2 and 5 million variations in the letters, or nucleotides, of our genes, which makes us more complex than earthworms.

All your DNA does is code for proteins. Proteins not only make our cells and tissues and organs but also are the chemical messengers that regulate nearly everything in our bodies. Each gene is made up of a combination of three letters, such as ATC, which then translate into a specific protein by assembling individual amino acids in a specific order and structure.

Even more mind-blowing is the fact that contained within each cell is your entire genetic code, the instructions to create every single part of your body and biology. The cells in your eye contain all the information needed to become bone or muscle or liver. How does your eye know to just be an eye?

The *epigenome.*

Your epigenome. This is the key to understanding how to unlock the secrets of healthy aging and longevity. Human DNA is the hardware and can't be changed (except with gene editing). The software that runs our life program is the epigenome, which provides instructions to the hardware on what to do. What is the epigenome? Think of it as the keys on your computer keyboard or the keys of a piano. Want to type the word "love" on your computer? You need to enter *L-O-V-E* on your keyboard. Your keyboard can create gibberish or a Nobel Prize–winning novel or the greatest love poem in history. A piano can create millions of different songs and types of music, from Mozart to reggae to rock to jazz to folk. It all depends on the inputs. Same keys, different results. Your DNA is no different. Your eye, for example, turns off all the genes that make every other organ, and just expresses the part of your DNA (or codes for the proteins) needed to become an optimally functioning eye cell. This is great news because it means we can modify our gene expression—which genes get turned on or off, which story we write in our book of life. A story of disability and disease, or a story of vitality, health, and longevity.

The Human Genome Project was one of science's greatest achievements, but everyone expected that it would unlock the secrets of and cures for disease. How did that turn out? Not so well. Yes, we learned a lot, but most chronic diseases, like heart disease, cancer, diabetes, and dementia, are not the result of a single or even a dozen genes. They are the downstream consequences of changes to your epigenome. It turns out that disease and biological aging are coding problems, instances where there is "corrupt" code in our operating systems. Even though we cannot change our genes (except through gene-editing tools like CRISPR), the fantastic news is that we can change our epigenome, or the coding problem. How? *DNA methylation*—something we have more control over than you would guess.

DNA methylation. DNA methylation is the single most important process controlling your epigenome. Chemical compounds called *methyl groups,* one carbon and three hydrogen molecules (CH_3), wrap around your DNA. These tiny little ubiquitous chemical groups literally control the function of your DNA by telling your body to either activate or silence a gene. The process of DNA methylation is highly influenced by your habits and environment, and it changes throughout your life for better or worse depending on the inputs to your body. It is those changes that help determine your biological age. When methyl groups are added to your DNA, the genes are silenced, or turned off. Similarly, when methyl groups are removed, the genes are turned on.

Methylation also regulates DNA protein production and repair, expression of genetic variations, hormones, metabolism, neurotransmitters, detoxification, and energy production. Many enzymes regulate methylation, and those vary greatly from person to person. These enzymes depend on helpers, coenzymes known as methylation factors. Thankfully we get most of these from food, including folate, vitamins B_6 and B_{12}, choline, trimethyl glycine, and more. But many of us have variations in our genes that require more or special forms of these methylating nutrients.

DNA methylation is highly influenced by your diet, exercise, stress, relationships, thoughts, nutritional status, toxins, sleep, infections, pretty much everything washing over us as we live our lives. Think of the process of DNA methylation (adding or taking away methyl groups, or CH_3) as keystrokes on a piano that change the song played — or how the epigenome translates its effects to the DNA. A single meal or a simple run can change your epigenetic marks by affecting the location of the methyl groups on the DNA or which keys of your piano get played. Even cuddling impacts your DNA methylation![3] Babies who don't get enough love and affection are known to have developmental delays and lower IQ — all influenced by changes to their epigenome.[4] Your epigenetics can be positively or negatively influenced at every stage of life. The key is learning what optimizes DNA methylation for health and longevity and shuts down disease. For example, you want the genes for inflammation turned off, while genes that suppress tumors are turned on. That is what you will learn — how to live and be in a way that rewrites your book of life, a story that is full of abundant energy, vibrant health, and a long, active, disease-free existence.

Methylation: A Short Guide

To illustrate the profound impact of epigenetic changes, we need to look no further than a landmark experiment by epigeneticist Randy Jirtle. His team experimented with two groups of genetically identical agouti mice, special mice bred to be yellow, fat, and diabetic. They gave one group methylation factors, including vitamin B_6, folate, B_{12}, choline, and genistein (a soy-derived phytochemical), and the other the normal mouse chow. They then bred the mice, and the offspring were dramatically different. The offspring of the group that received the methylation support were born brown, thin, and healthy![5]

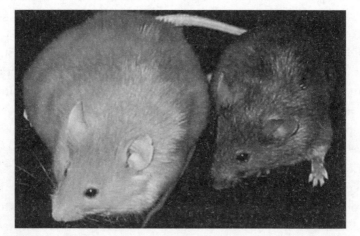

Photo courtesy of Dana Dolinoy (University of Michigan) and Randy Jirtle (Duke University)

A picture is worth a thousand words. Remember, these mice are genetically identical. The only change was a few vitamins and soy phytonutrients, which changed the instructions for the DNA methyl groups, determining which genetic variations turned on or off.[6]

Imagine if we modified our habits to turn on all the right genes and turn down the expression of the harmful ones. The result: a long health span and life span. The reason I am taking you down this scientific rabbit hole is to help you understand biological aging and how to reverse it.

The overarching concept here is simple. Our genes are fixed. But the genes that are *expressed* in our book of life, which genes are turned on or off, genes of health and vitality or genes of disease and early death, are modifiable. It turns out that more than 90 percent of chronic disease is determined not by our genome but by our *"exposome."*[7] Conversely, that means that 90 percent of our health and our potential for longevity results not from our inherited genetic code but from the exposures that influence our genes.

THE EXPOSOME: THE KEY TO UNLOCKING HEALTH AND LONGEVITY

What is the exposome?

It is everything that has happened to you over your lifetime and even what has happened to you in utero or to your ancestors that is imprinted in your epigenome. The trauma of your ancestors is imprinted in their epigenome, and it gets passed on to you. Descendants of concentration camp survivors have their parents' or grandparents' trauma imprinted on their genes. The result: They can literally inherit PTSD, anxiety, and depression. Data from multiple studies proves this.[8] And not only emotional trauma is inherited. Animal studies show that exposure to glyphosate, a toxic weed killer used on 70 percent of crops, in grandparents can cause disease in their grandchildren who have never been exposed.[9]

Every input influences our epigenome—every bite of food, exercise or lack of exercise, stress, loneliness, toxins, allergens, microbes, our microbiome, our thoughts, feelings, and relationships. Every sadness, every joy. Your senses, your metabolism, the trillions of microbes living in your gut, every chemical exposure, every sunset watched or argument had is registered in real time within your biology and regu-lates all the switches that control your health, your epigenome. *The exposome regulates the epigenome.* Your state of health or disease and your biological age are the result of life washing over your genes. And the good news is we have an enormous ability to change those inputs.

We can eat whole real food, move our bodies, cut our toxic envi-ronmental exposures, heal our traumas, change our thinking and mindset, build community and love in our lives. And these are just first-order interventions. The rapidly progressing science of healthy aging gives us many new "hacks" to improve our epigenome, includ-ing supplements, medications, and other novel treatments like *hormesis* (stress that doesn't kill you but makes you stronger, like fasting or cold plunges). Although we are less than a decade into the era of measuring our epigenetic biological clocks, a few small but important studies have shown that we can literally reverse our biological age through simple interventions.

Steve Horvath and his colleagues gave a group of adults three com-pounds thought to help with longevity: human growth hormone, DHEA (an adrenal hormone that declines with age), and metformin (a diabetes drug that may have longevity benefits). While I prefer that we use nature-made compounds when possible, certain medications may play a role in treating abnormal aging. What they found in this study astounded them. They expected that perhaps they could slow the biological clock slightly, but they found that they had reduced the biological age of participants by about two and a half years, after a year of treatment, a change that persisted even six months after they stopped treatment.[10]

Another study in a typically vitamin D–deficient population found that taking 4,000 IU of vitamin D_3 could reduce biological age by 1.85 years in just sixteen weeks.[11] Yet one more study on Polish women showed that a Mediterranean diet could lower biological age by 1.47 years over the course of a year.[12] Their chronological age increased by a year while their biological age reversed.

Dr Kara Fitzgerald and her colleagues found even more remarkable results in a study of forty-three healthy adult men between fifty and seventy-two using a comprehensive functional medicine lifestyle intervention. They followed an eight-week treatment program that included a whole foods phytochemical-rich, anti-inflammatory, methylation-supporting diet (an upgrade from the Mediterranean diet), exercise, sleep optimization, stress reduction (breathing techniques), probiotics, and a fruit and vegetable phytonutrient powder with phytochemicals known to improve methylation. The treatment group reversed their biological clock (measured by DNA methylation) by an incredible 3.23 years in just eight weeks compared to the control group.[13] Though it was a small study, the results were statistically significant and, frankly, very exciting.

Imagine if those changes and other known interventions were combined over many years. How much younger would we be able to become? While the research on the use of the DNA methylation biological clock is in its infancy, it opens the door to an accurate tool that can measure the effects of various interventions on longevity and health. The younger our biology, the healthier we are, the more youthful we feel, the longer we live.

Chapter 4

The Ten Hallmarks of Aging

It is a magnificent feeling to recognize the unity of a complex of phenomena which appear to be things quite apart from the direct visible truth.

— Albert Einstein

Much longevity research has focused on the underlying common pathways or mechanisms of aging but not necessarily the causes. The goal is to discover tools, therapies, and technologies that will prevent, repair, or renew our biology to reverse the hallmarks of aging. But these hallmarks are not individual separate phenomena; they interact in a complex integrated network—each influencing and being influenced by others. Each hallmark is affected by various imbalances—too much or too little of certain inputs that can negatively impact the expression and progression of the hallmark. Understanding those interactions and weblike connections is the key to solving the puzzle of aging. What drives these hallmarks, these biochemical and genetic dysfunctions that manifest as disease and accelerated aging? And more importantly, what can we do to create balance and slow or even reverse the progression of the hallmarks of aging? First, let's dive into the ten hallmarks of aging themselves so we can understand what can go wrong when our systems experience imbalance. Then in Part II, we get to the fun stuff: exactly what you can do to create balance, live more energetically and youthfully, and extend your health span and life span.

HALLMARK 1: DISRUPTED HORMONE AND NUTRIENT
SIGNALING—FOOD AND AGING

The wondrous nature of human biology is revealed in the beautiful complexity, interdependence, and coordinated nature of the biochemical systems that sustain life. Things go wrong when we deviate from living in harmony with nature or in balance with ourselves and our environment. Disease and accelerated aging are not mistakes. They are our body's best attempt to deal with a bad set of circumstances. Health and longevity are our natural states, but only if we understand how our bodies are designed to work best. We have evolved extraordinary nutrient-sensing pathways that are essential to understand how to eat to avoid disease, activate robust health, and live for a long time. When these pathways are dysregulated, aging accelerates.

Years ago, I went to a longevity conference at the Menla center in upstate New York that brought together leading researchers in aging, Nobel Prize winners, and Tibetan doctors and the Dalai Lama. I met Lenny Guarente there, the MIT scientist who, along with Dr David Sinclair, demonstrated dramatic life extension in yeast and mice even in the absence of calorie restriction, previously the only proven way to extend life in animal models (at least in the lab). They used *resveratrol,* the phytochemical in red wine, to activate the *sirtuin pathway;* sirtuins are proteins that regulate several essential biological repair processes. But before you stock up on red wine, you should know that they gave the mice the equivalent of 1,500 bottles.

On the way to a talk, I asked him the about the causes of aging and how the sirtuins are regulated, and what impairs their life-extending activity. He simply said, "Sugar!"

Our bodies have exquisite mechanisms for sampling the environment, for sensing the levels of nutrients—amino acids, sugars, and fatty acids. From moment to moment they modify a myriad of chemical reactions that trigger either *autophagy*—the process of cellular recycling and cleanup—or *protein synthesis,* making new proteins and parts. Breakdown or buildup. How do our bodies know what to do?

We have four key nutrient-sensing systems that work together, with overlapping redundancies designed to beautifully protect us from disease and abnormal aging: *insulin and insulin signaling, mTOR, AMPK,* and *sirtuins.* Most of the dietary and lifestyle strategies that prevent disease, promote health, and extend life work through these nutrient-sensing systems. Understanding the *why* of aging will help you make sense of the *what,* the strategies and tools in the Young Forever Program that incorporate all this science into practical daily approaches for health and longevity.

Our modern diet and way of living interfere with these systems. They evolved in a very different time—a time of food scarcity, not abundance, a time of profound nutritional density in our food supply, a time of natural movement and exercise, a time of rhythmic living in harmony with day and night and the cycles of nature, a time of few toxins and none of the modern stresses of life. For example, we evolved in a symbiotic relationship with our diet, which comprised 800 species of wild plants. These are nearly absent in our modern diet, which is comprised of primarily four crops (corn, wheat, soy, and rice), things never consumed by our hunter-gatherer ancestors. Our ancestors' diet was phytochemically rich and contained ten times as much fiber and dramatically higher levels of vitamins, minerals, omega-3 fats, and phytochemicals.[1] Our cells and biochemical pathways are dependent on these coevolutionary raw materials. The absence of this nutrient-rich diet ages and kills us quickly.

So how can we think about these nutrient-sensing systems? How do we engage them in the right way at the right times to generate health? This will get a bit technical, but bear with me.

The Insulin-Signaling Pathway

For most of the 200,000 years that Homo sapiens have roamed the Earth, sugar was scarce and refined grains nonexistent. Other than an occasional late summer wild berry patch or beehive, humans have not been exposed to much sugar—maybe 22 teaspoons of something sweet a year. Today Americans eat 22 teaspoons a day (more than two 12-ounce/375-ml fizzy drinks), with kids eating more than 34 teaspoons a day (three and a half fizzy drinks a day). Sugar consumption has increased from 10 pounds (4.5 kg) per person a year in 1800 to 152 pounds (69 kg) per person each year. The honey hunters of Nepal climbed 100-foot trees with a burning bush to gather honey. Imagine if every time you wanted a cookie you had to climb a tree with a burning bush. The invention of the flour mill in the 1800s flooded our diet with refined starches. The advent of post–World War II industrial agriculture focused on producing an abundance of starchy calories to feed a growing hungry world worked. The development of dwarf wheat, containing the super-starch amylopectin A, which has a higher glycemic index than table sugar, made a bad situation worse. Now the average American consumes 133 pounds (60 kg) of flour a year. Below the neck your body doesn't know the difference between a fizzy drink and a bagel.

What is the consequence of this flood of starch and sugar over our 200,000-year-old evolutionary survival pathways? I already mentioned how it damages your DNA. We have hundreds of genes that help us adapt to scarcity and starvation and very few that help us handle abundance, otherwise known as the pharmacologic megadoses of sugar and starch flooding our system every day. Our bodies are elegantly designed not only to navigate the stress of not enough food, but also to build new cells and tissues and structures when food is abundant. It's the dance between scarcity and abundance that is the key to health and longevity.

It turns out the longevity switches are regulated by the timing, the quality, and the amount of nutrients in our diet—primarily the carbohydrates and sugars, and the amino acids in protein. Much of longevity research is focused on how to properly regulate these longevity switches. Food is the master controller, the conductor of these longevity pathways. Not just protein, carbs, and fats but also the 25,000 *phytochemicals* (plant-signaling molecules), many of which act beneficially on these longevity switches. While current science may not consider these essential nutrients, they are, in fact, *essential*. A lack of these nutrients may not cause an immediate deficiency disease like scurvy from lack of vitamin C, but they cause long-latency deficiency diseases — heart disease, cancer, diabetes, dementia, and accelerated aging.

If I were to prescribe one intervention to extend life, to prevent and reverse chronic disease, it would be to dramatically reduce or eliminate sugar and refined starch from your diet. The flood of sugar and starch drives your pancreas to produce more and more insulin to keep blood sugar under control. This leads to insulin resistance, or the inability of our cells to "hear" the signals from insulin. What does the body do then? It produces more and more insulin. Unfortunately, this excessive amount of insulin drives sugar and fat into the cells, primarily into the fat cells around your abdominal organs — visceral fat, otherwise known as belly fat — locks the fat in those cells, slows down metabolism, and increases hunger and craving for carbohydrates, all things that worsen blood sugar control and insulin resistance and lead to the diseases of aging.

Dr Jorge Plutzky, the head of preventive cardiology at Harvard, once said that if you could find a group of centenarians with perfectly clean arteries, they would have one thing in common — they would be insulin-sensitive.

High levels of sugar and starch don't just act through the insulin-signaling pathway; they adversely affect all the longevity switches, including the mTOR, AMPK, and sirtuin pathways. Bottom line: The most important thing you can do for healthy aging is to balance your blood sugar and keep your insulin levels low and your cells insulin-sensitive, which means eating a low-sugar, low-starch diet with plenty of good-quality fats and protein, and a boatload of phytochemical- and fiber-rich fruits and vegetables.

The Secret of Autophagy: Regulating mTOR and Self-Cannibalism

mTOR is important for regulating cell growth, protein synthesis, mitochondrial function, cell senescence (programmed cell death), and more. Low levels of glucose and amino acids in the blood signal danger or scarcity and inhibit this key longevity switch called the mammalian/mechanistic target of rapamycin (mTOR). With mTOR, we want it sometimes on and other times off. For example, we want mTOR turned on when we are exercising, building muscle and creating new proteins, but we want it off to enhance autophagy and cellular cleanup and repair.

Autophagy, which literally means "self-eating," is a recycling system that is essential to our biology. It is a built-in ancient survival mechanism. It cleans out old proteins, damaged cells, and other gunk that we don't want accumulating in our bodies. The old proteins and cell parts get carried to a *lysosome.* Imagine a little Pac-Man, like a vacuum cleaner, that goes around finding all the old and damaged proteins and engulfs them, digests them, and breaks them apart into their component amino acids, which are then reused in the building of new proteins.

Without autophagy, we accumulate debris, the equivalent of dumping garbage in your garbage can and never emptying it. There are many ways to keep this process of breakdown and rebuilding turned on and turned off at the right times so we can make new proteins and build muscle, but also recycle old cells and clean up unwanted gunk.

Without regular periods of autophagy, these diseases can take hold:

- Alzheimer's
- Atherosclerosis (leading to heart attack and stroke)
- Fatty liver disease
- Obesity
- Cancer
- Parkinson's
- Polycystic kidney disease
- Polycystic ovarian syndrome
- Type 2 diabetes

Some believe we should limit protein (especially animal protein) and amino acids to silence mTOR and activate autophagy. The data, to be fair, is confusing. A constant influx of nutrients keeps mTOR on. However, when mTOR is silenced for long periods, we can't create new proteins or build muscle.

The loss of muscle (sarcopenia) is one of the key accelerators of rapid aging and disease. Unless we have adequate high-quality protein with the right amino acids, found primarily in animal protein, as we age we lose muscle and replace our youthful, strong, low-fat fillet steak muscle with weak, fat-infused Wagyu rib eye. This results in impaired glucose metabolism and insulin resistance, higher stress hormones (e.g., cortisol), lower growth hormone (needed for healing and repair), lower testosterone, and increased inflammation, which can all lead to increased weakness, disability, increased hospitalization, immobility, and loss of independence.

Cycling periods of fasting or caloric restriction (which silences mTOR) with periods of adequate high-quality protein (which activates mTOR) to maintain and build new muscle is a powerful strategy for healthy aging. But not only do amino acids activate mTOR; glucose and sugars activate it too, and not in a good way. Overactivation of mTOR by sugar and starch can cause cancer.[2]

The key is to give your body a break from the constant influx of calories on a regular basis. And to ensure the highest-quality nutrient intake that is low in sugar and starch, high in good fats and phytochemical-rich vegetables and fruit, and high in quality protein to activate protein synthesis. Regular exercise, especially vigorous high-intensity interval training, also activates autophagy. There are certain phytonutrients that mimic a condition of beneficial stress called *hormesis* (discussed in Chapter 7), which can activate autophagy too. These include the polyphenols in coffee, oleuropein in extra virgin olive oil, resveratrol in red grape skin, catechins in green tea, turmeric, berberine, and a gut metabolite from phytochemicals in pomegranate called urolithin A.

Rapamycin: Silencing mTOR with Medication

Is there a way to activate autophagy by mimicking fasting without fasting? Rapamycin could be an answer. It is a molecule found on Easter Island in the 1960s by a group of scientists looking for medicinal compounds. The island is also called Rapa Nui, a place of mysterious giant statues that defy earthly explanation. From the back of one of the statues, scientists scraped off what may turn out to be the fountain of youth. At first, the compound was thought to be a good antifungal, but research was shelved for years until scientists discovered its immune-modulating properties, which led to its use in preventing organ-transplant rejection. Then it was discovered to silence the mTOR pathway, mimicking fasting and optimizing this longevity switch and autophagy.

Many longevity hackers have started to take low-dose rapamycin based on preliminary studies. It cannot be taken daily, but if used, for example, three days a week for five weeks with eight weeks off it may have most of the benefits without risks. Lower intermittent doses can avert some of the side effects, but longevity researchers are working on *rapalogues,* or analogs of rapamycin without side effects. Soon we will have medication to help us induce autophagy, one of the most essential pathways to preventing and reversing disease and extending healthy life span.

The elegant nutrient-sensing systems in our body are listening for signals of scarcity or abundance, and through a whole cascade of biochemical reactions, they adapt to what's needed in the moment. The key to health and longevity is balance: activating these pathways enough to rebuild and heal and grow but not too much to cause damage.

AMPK: The Sweetness of Long Life

AMP-activated protein kinase (AMPK) is a critical enzyme found in every mammalian cell. It's activated during times of "good" stress, called hormesis (discussed in Chapter 10), like when you are exercising, fasting, or engaging in caloric restriction. These enzymes sense low levels of energy in the body. Just as your car runs on petrol, your cells run on ATP (adenosine triphosphate), your main energy source. ATP molecules give away one or two of their phosphate molecules to fuel your cells. That turns the ATP molecule into ADP or AMP (adenosine di- or monophosphate). The AMPK enzyme detects this dip in energy supply, activating the enzyme to do its work.

What happens when it is turned on? Everything you need to reverse disease and increase a healthy life span.[3] It improves your cells' ability to produce energy, reverses insulin resistance and improves blood sugar control, enhances stress resistance, and improves your cells' housekeeping functions.

As we age, AMPK becomes less sensitive to low levels of energy and nutrients, meaning it turns on less, leading to a slower metabolism and increased oxidative stress and preventing autophagy. These changes activate your ancient immune system to turn on, creating more inflammation, which in turn further impedes AMPK. A vicious cycle! But a fixable one with the right diet, lifestyle, supplements, and even medications.

Metformin: A Potential Fountain of Youth

A very popular, widely prescribed, inexpensive type 2 diabetes medication called metformin, which works in part by activating AMPK, discovered in 1957, has recently caught the attention of aging researchers as a potential drug therapy for the underlying pathways involved in disease and aging.[4] Though the jury is still out on its overall impact on aging and long-term side effects, it holds potential as a compound that may modulate the nutrient-sensing pathways, especially AMPK, in ways that slow or even reverse aging. In animal models it prevents cancer and heart disease. In population studies (which can't prove cause and effect) metformin reduces age-related disease, including cancer, cardiovascular disease, and dementia, and lowers mortality in diabetics taking it compared to nondiabetics not taking it. Is there a catch? Maybe.

A large experiment known as the Diabetes Prevention Program (DPP), involving more than 1,079 pre-diabetic participants, studied the effects of lifestyle versus metformin versus a control group without any interventions.[5] While the metformin reduced the progression to type 2 diabetes by 31 percent, the lifestyle intervention reduced it by 58 percent. The study was done in the early 2000s when low-fat diets were still believed to be the key to weight loss, and the key dietary intervention in the study was fat restriction. The other lifestyle interventions, including exercise, education, and group support, may have been a large part of the benefit seen. Even though we know that low-fat diets are, in fact, not helpful and may be harmful for type 2 diabetes, the study still showed that lifestyle was much more effective than metformin in reducing progression to type 2 diabetes.

We know now that high-carbohydrate diets, even from grains and beans, can be problematic for diabetics (and for anyone overweight) because they stimulate the insulin-signaling pathways. The carbohydrate-insulin hypothesis of weight gain and diabetes has been well established by David Ludwig at Harvard and others.[6] Any diet high in starch or sugar that stimulates insulin will promote weight gain and diabetes.

Conversely, the work of Dr Sarah Hallberg and others has shown clearly that high-fat ketogenic diets can not only prevent but completely reverse advanced type 2 diabetes in 60 percent of cases, and can also eliminate the need for most diabetes medications and insulin injections and result in significant weight loss compared to high-carbohydrate diets.[7] And all the impacts on cholesterol and heart disease risk factors were positive.[8] So if a diet low in fat, along with basic lifestyle changes, can reduce progression to diabetes by 58 percent, what could a low-insulin-producing (higher-fat, low-carb, moderate-protein) diet do to prevent diabetes? The answer: a lot! And perhaps far more than metformin can achieve.

The question really is not what drug is best to lower the onslaught of age-related disease linked to our high-carb, high-sugar, and high-calorie diet, but what is the best diet and lifestyle intervention that will create the same or a better result. While metformin may turn out to be a useful tool for longevity, it is not the first place I would start. There are many ways to activate AMPK and the longevity pathways, including time-restricted eating, fasting, exercise, heat therapy, and phytochemicals. Many plant compounds have been found to activate AMPK and may result in longevity benefits similar to those of metformin, including areca nut, saffron, berberine from goldenseal, aloe, resveratrol, ginseng, reishi, hot peppers, artemisia, black cumin seed, bitter melon, tangerines, chlorogenic acid from coffee, and capsaicin from peppers.[9]

For now, I prefer to focus on the hallmarks of aging by addressing the root causes of those hallmarks and by using the lifestyle and other non-pharmacologic approaches featured in the Young Forever Program. But you may want to experiment with metformin after consultation with your doctor, especially if you have insulin resistance.

Sirtuins: Yeast, Wine, and Longevity

While we may think that simple organisms like yeast or mice can't tell us much about human biology, they do. Biological organisms arose from the same primordial soup billions of years ago and have many of the same genes and metabolic pathways. Discoveries by Leonard Guarente[10] and Dr David Sinclair at MIT in the 1990s helped us understand a key pathway that regulates aging and disease: *sirtuins*.[11]

Sirtuins are a family of signaling proteins that regulate gene transcription (the making of new proteins), lower inflammation and oxidative stress, and improve metabolism and cellular energy production.[12] They are key players in the health of our mitochondria. In short, our energy production depends on sirtuins. They are also essential for fixing DNA damage throughout the body and protecting our telomeres.

Sirtuins are critical to making us more insulin-sensitive. They detect low-nutrient states (e.g., when we're fasting) and kick in all the benefits noted earlier. However, dumping pounds of sugar and flour on these sirtuins essentially prevents them from doing their job. And we keep eating more sugar and starch because they are biologically addictive, creating a vicious cycle of disease and rapid aging.[13]

As we age, sirtuin activity decreases along with all the sirtuins' beneficial effects. Increasing their activity is key to a long, healthy life.

What turns sirtuins on? Remarkably, nature has provided myriad ways to increase the activity of sirtuins. The remarkable world of phytochemicals contains virtual elixirs of health and youth. The Rockefeller Foundation is spending $200 million to analyze the 25,000 medicinal compounds found in the plant kingdom.[14] Food is medicine. And the right medicine at the right dose and the right time can help us live long, healthy, vibrant lives.

As I've mentioned, early studies found that resveratrol from red grape skin activates the sirtuin pathway.[15] But remember, the dose was the equivalent of 1,500 bottles of red wine. Enjoy a glass of red wine occasionally, but don't expect it to extend your life! Other beneficial compounds are proanthocyanidins, found in berries; quercetin, found in onions; curcumin, from turmeric; catechins, from green tea; persimmon; kaempferol, found in cruciferous vegetables; oligonol, from lychee fruit; butein, found in the Chinese lacquer tree and many flowering plants; and many compounds, like paeonol, used in traditional Chinese medicine. Even certain medications, like metformin and melatonin, may work in part by their effects on the sirtuins.

In addition to plant compounds, diet and lifestyle play a profound role in effectively activating the sirtuin pathway. A low-sugar, low-starch diet rich in plants and phytochemicals, like that described in *The Pegan Diet,* is the foundation of activating sirtuins. A fizzy drink or bagel is the best way to turn off their benefits. Periods of dietary restriction (a 14- to 16-hour daily fast) and longer fasts are also effective.

How does our body naturally activate sirtuins? It makes a compound called *nicotinamide adenine dinucleotide (NAD+).* NAD+ is key to energy production in the cells. But it also activates DNA repair, inhibits inflammation, improves your cells' ability to handle stress, increases new brain connections or neuroplasticity, and optimizes mitochondrial function—all things necessary to a healthy and long life. Unfortunately, NAD+ production decreases as we age. In Chapter 15 we will dive deeper into how to boost your NAD+ levels. It is among the most exciting potential therapies for longevity. Regular aerobic exercise also activates sirtuins. In fact, many of exercise's known benefits for health and longevity are due to its action on the sirtuin pathway. Exercise also stimulates a key enzyme called NAMPT, which is needed to produce more NAD+.

NAD+, NMN, NR: The Alphabet Soup of Youthfulness

David Sinclair, PhD, author of *Lifespan: Why We Age—and Why We Don't Have To,* and his colleagues at Harvard have pioneered much of the research surrounding NAD+ and sirtuin activity. NAD+ is derived from niacin, or vitamin B_3. It is a key part of the body's energy (ATP) production system in the mitochondria but has more far-reaching effects, including all the downstream benefits of activating the sirtuin pathway for cellular health, DNA repair, and longevity. It is produced in the body in a few steps from NR (nicotinamide riboside) and then NMN (nicotinamide mononucleotide), both of which are being researched as supplements that increase NAD+ levels in the body. These compounds have shown powerful protective effects against disease and aging. In a fascinating conversation I had with Dr Sinclair, he told me an anecdotal story about giving older mice NAD+ boosters in his lab. These compounds gave the old mice so much energy that they literally broke the mouse treadmill, which wasn't designed to have mice run for 3 kilometers! Young mice can barely run for 1 kilometer without pooping out. NAD+ has even reversed "mousopause," restoring fertility to older female mice.[16]

NAD+ plays a critical role in regulating our metabolism and circadian rhythm via the sirtuins. It decreases with age, which means less sirtuin activity. Supplementation of NAD+ and NAD+ precursors NR and NMN have been able to restore youthful levels, reversing age-related pathology and extending life. It is something I take every day, along with many other top aging researchers. NAD+ (and precursors NR and NMN) may be one of the most powerful discoveries in healthy life extension— it may be as close to the fountain of youth as we can get.[17]

Dysfunctional nutrient-sensing pathways (insulin signaling, mTOR, AMPK, and sirtuins) are the most critical hallmark of aging. Food is the key lever to either harm (with our modern diet) or optimize these pathways. The bottom line: Cut the sugar and starch and processed food. Eat lots of phytochemicals from colorful fruits and vegetables, good fats, and high-quality protein. Engage in good stress that activates these pathways, including exercise and potentially longer fasts. And give yourself breaks from eating by leaving at least 12 to 14 hours between dinner and breakfast (more to come on intermittent fasting and time-restricted eating in Chapter 14).

HALLMARK 2: DNA DAMAGE AND MUTATIONS—PROBLEMS WITH OUR GENETIC BLUEPRINT

Damage to our DNA is one of the hallmarks of aging. How does our DNA get damaged? Each day our DNA gets up to 100,000 little hits, death by a thousand cuts—damage by UV radiation, environmental toxins, our nutrient-depleted, high-sugar, processed-food diet, and other stressors. The accumulation of these insults accelerates aging. Thankfully we have built-in repair systems that seek out damaged DNA and fix it. That is a key job of the sirtuins. But even if 99 percent of damage is reversed, the remaining 1 percent accumulates over our lifetime. Our cells also divide, and that means re-creating the DNA blueprint in each cell. Over your lifetime your DNA produces 10 quadrillion copies of itself through cell division. Sometimes there are glitches in the copy machine, and our DNA blueprint is reproduced with these glitches. Think of these as typos in your book of life.

What can be done about this? By avoiding DNA-damaging insults (eliminating processed foods and limiting toxins, radiation, and stressors the best you can) and activating our repair systems with the Young Forever Program—and eventually editing our genes through tools like CRISPR—we can go in and repair the accumulated insults and damage to our DNA.

HALLMARK 3: TELOMERE SHORTENING—BECOMING UNRAVELED

Our telomeres, the little caps at the end of our chromosomes, shorten as we age and eventually can't hold the tightly protected DNA double helix to prevent it from unraveling. Each time cells replicate, the caps are removed so the DNA can be read, but the telomere shortens a little bit until it is so short the cell stops dividing or commits programmed cell death (also known as *apoptosis*). This is a normal consequence of cell division. The longer our telomeres, the more years of healthy DNA replication we have. The shorter they are, the shorter our life. Also, sometimes the cells don't die but turn into zombie cells (see hallmark 6) spewing out inflammatory compounds that accelerate aging.

The good news is that we have tremendous influence over our telomeres. The usual lifestyle transgressions shorten them—our toxic processed diet, sugar, environmental toxins, sedentary lifestyle, and psychological stress. Shorter telomeres are linked to all the problems of aging and increase the risk of not just gray hair, but heart disease, cancer, immune dysfunction, and more. A whole foods phytonutrient-rich diet, exercise, meditation, sleep, love, and even a multivitamin all lengthen the telomeres.

HALLMARK 4: DAMAGED PROTEINS—MALFORMED, MISSHAPEN, DYSFUNCTIONAL MOLECULES

Remember that all DNA does is code for proteins. These proteins regulate everything in your body. Your organs, tissues, and cells are made from proteins. Your cellular messenger molecules, like hormones, peptides, immune molecules, and neurotransmitters, are made from proteins. Proteins form your information superhighway, facilitating trillions of chemical signals and reactions each second. Many messenger proteins that contain the instructions for life are often short-lived. And they can be damaged by all the same insults that damage DNA. The function of your proteins is determined not only by their amino acid sequence but also by their three-dimensional shape and their complex folding patterns. If those proteins are damaged and misshapen, they don't work.

Thankfully we have a built-in recycling system called *autophagy*, referred to in hallmark 1—remember the little Pac-Man lysosome that engulfs gunk and cleans out our cells? It's a brilliant system. Yet most of us live in ways that thwart that system. We are constantly consuming calories. This endless stream of food (starch, sugar, and protein) activates mTOR, which shuts down autophagy. We never give our bodies the much-needed break from the flood of energy needed to do the cleanup and repair work. Periods of fasting (even overnight for 12 hours) give our body a chance to clean up the messes and damaged proteins we create from the way we live.

Sugar and Starch

In addition to the vicissitudes of life causing natural damage to proteins and DNA, we are amid a terrible crisis of sugar and starch overload, the worst culprit. When too much sugar or starch is coursing through your bloodstream and tissues, it gloms onto proteins, causing irreversible damage called *glycation*. Think of the crackling surface of crème brûlée, or crispy chicken skin or the crust of a baguette. Known as the browning or Maillard reaction between amino acids and sugars, this is what makes food taste good. However, in your body this reaction produces *AGEs* (*advanced glycation end products*) that bind to *RAGEs* (*receptors for advanced glycation end products*). And they do exactly what their acronyms suggest—they cause your body to age and rage against the insult of too much sugar and starch. Once the sugars bind to the proteins, they become dysfunctional and cause disease.

The test doctors use to assess blood sugar control measures *hemoglobin A1c,* the result of sugars combining with the hemoglobin in your red blood cells. But this doesn't just happen in your blood. Damaged collagen leads to aging skin and bones, glycation in your eyes results in cataracts, and blood vessels stiffen, resulting in high blood pressure, heart failure, kidney disease, and dementia, often called type 3 diabetes.

It turns out that this load of sugar and starch is the most powerful driver of aging. It both shuts off the longevity switches and accelerates nearly all the hallmarks of aging, shortening our telomeres and damaging our DNA, proteins, epigenome, mitochondria, and microbiome. Sugar and starch also drive accelerated inflammation, create hormonal chaos, and age our stem cells. If you want to live a long and healthy life, sugar and starch should be either eliminated or used very occasionally.

HALLMARK 5: EPIGENETIC DAMAGE—A DYSFUNCTIONAL PIANO PLAYER

Remember the science of epigenetics? The piano player plays the keys of our DNA, producing a melody that is health or cacophony that is disease. Think of the epigenome as a very sensitive microphone picking up healing or harmful signals from your environment. Similarly, your DNA, through the epigenome, is listening carefully to all the messages conveyed by your whole life. Too much bad stuff damages the epigenome and makes you age faster, and the good stuff translates into instructions for your genetic code. The wonder of this discovery is that though our DNA is fixed, the epigenome—*how* the music of your life is played—is not; it is highly influenced by things under our control, like our exposome (and even some things out of our control, like environmental toxins and radiation).

The longevity tools and strategies in *Young Forever* work in part by exerting a positive influence on the epigenome.

HALLMARK 6: SENESCENT CELLS—THE ATTACK OF THE ZOMBIE CELLS

The zombie apocalypse is real, but it's not the kind you imagine. As we've discussed, programmed cellular death, or *apoptosis,* clears out old or damaged cells and recycles parts for new cells. But sometimes cells don't quite die. They become *zombie cells* or *senescent cells.* Zombie cells are caused by DNA damage, critically short telomeres, and chemical or toxic stress, including our inflammatory diet and lifestyle. They accelerate all the age-related diseases: cancer, heart disease, liver disease, dementia, Parkinson's, cataracts, arthritis, and muscle loss, or sarcopenia.

While zombie cells wander around your body, they secrete dangerous molecules called *cytokines* and other molecules that drive inflammation and cause neighboring cells to become senescent, or zombie, cells too (which continues the cascade). And as we age, immune-system functioning wanes, making this cycle worse. The inflammatory messages secreted by those cells flood your body, causing damage, or "inflammaging" (see hallmark 10). Inflammation drives the formation of even more zombie cells, a dangerous, deadly, self-perpetuating cycle.

Much aging research is focused on how we kill these zombie cells. Luckily, there are natural and pharmaceutical compounds that can kill them, stop the progression of inflammaging, and allow for tissue repair, rejuvenation, and remodeling. These are called *senolytics,* a new category of natural and pharmaceutical compounds.

One study combined *quercetin,* a natural compound found in apples and onions, with a leukemia chemotherapy drug called *dasatinib* to kill zombie cells; life span in mice was extended by 36 percent.[18] Other natural compounds have been found to kill zombie cells too. The edible plant kingdom contains 25,000 different *phytochemicals,* molecules produced by plants that help defend them from harsh conditions and predators. Remarkably, most of these compounds directly regulate many human biological functions and systems. I believe we coevolved with plants to borrow their medicines to keep us healthy. I call this *symbiotic phytoadaptation.*

Senolytics include *fisetin,* from strawberries, persimmons, apples, cucumbers, and onions; *luteolin,* found in carrots, broccoli, artichokes, onions, chrysanthemum flowers, cabbages, and apple skins; *quercetin,* found in apples, grapes, berries, broccoli, citrus fruits, and cherries; *curcumin,* found in turmeric; and *piperlongumine,* an extract of goldenrod and an alkaloid found in long peppers.

It might soon be possible to take a supplement with the right combination of natural senolytics and even new pharmaceutical compounds that can arrest and reverse the zombie apocalypse. Other emerging longevity therapies such as hyperbaric oxygen therapy (see Chapter 10) can also kill zombie cells.

HALLMARK 7: DEPLETED ENERGY—THE DECLINE OF OUR MITOCHONDRIA

Ever marvel at the endless energy of a three-year-old bouncing around and hyperengaged? Now imagine a ninety-year-old behaving the same way. Not likely. Why? Energy. What explains the difference? Mitochondria.

These tiny ancient organelles combine food and oxygen to produce energy that runs everything in our body. They take in raw materials— fatty acids, sugars, amino acids, and oxygen—and run them through an assembly line that produces ATP (adenosine triphosphate), our body's fuel. Like our car engine, they also produce exhaust in the form of water (which we pee out), carbon dioxide (which we breathe out), and free radicals that need to be neutralized by antioxidants. It's a beautiful system, but one vulnerable to injury from an excess of calories, sugar, environmental toxins, stress, an imbalanced microbiome, infection, or anything that causes inflammation.

The difference between the three-year-old and the ninety-year-old is the number and state of their mitochondria. As we age, mitochondrial DNA mutations accumulate, free radicals increase, and mitochondria drop in number and functioning, especially as we lose muscle. Hence the decline in energy. Those who do not take care of their mitochondria or who have less of them are more likely to be frail and 50 percent more likely to die. In fact, mitochondrial dysfunction is found in nearly all age-related diseases, including diabetes, heart disease, cancer, dementia, and Parkinson's. It is now even understood to be at the root of mental illness and neurological disorders such as schizophrenia and autism.

The way we live and eat triggers a cascade of exhaust, of free radicals and *oxidative stress* (oxygen damage we know of as rusting, or as an apple turning brown, or as skin damage). But oxidation is not always a bad thing. A little bit of oxidation exerts a positive influence that signals danger and activates our ancient protective and defense systems. Unchecked oxidation is bad for you, but free radicals are also signaling molecules used by the immune system to fight infection and cancer. Reducing the overproduction of free radicals and upregulating our body's own antioxidant systems is a key part of keeping balance as we age.

The challenge is that we live in a world that is bad for mitochondria and produces unchecked oxidative stress: processed food, stress, toxic bugs in our microbiome, a plethora of toxic environmental chemicals, radiation, and a lifestyle where only 23 percent of Americans get the recommended amount of exercise. The mitochondria are the place where metabolism occurs, so considering 93 percent of Americans are metabolically unhealthy, more than nine out of ten

Americans have poorly functioning or not enough mitochondria.[19] But this is not inevitable.

The good news is we now know how to clean up and eliminate damaged mitochondria. And we can make more mitochondria and upgrade our engines to run far better, boosting our energy. It's like turning a sluggish 1970 Dodge Dart spewing toxic exhaust into a brand-new zippy, clean Tesla. The best way to clean up and rejuvenate old mitochondria is to eat a whole foods low-starch-and-sugar, good-fat, microbiome-supporting, polyphenol-rich diet, practice intermittent fasting or caloric restriction, and incorporate hormesis (good stress) routines like cold plunges or showers, aerobic exercise, strength training, and a few key supplements.

The Young Forever Program will lay out, step by step, food by food, activity by activity, how to activate mitochondrial repair and renewal, fix problems with your epigenome, kill zombie cells, repair your DNA, and lengthen your telomeres.

HALLMARK 8: OF MICROBES AND MEN—THE LINK BETWEEN GUT HEALTH AND LONGEVITY

Denis Burkitt, an Irish physician and medical missionary in Africa in the mid-twentieth century, first noticed the link between poop and health.[20] Observing the differences between tribal hunter-gatherer populations and their genetic cousins who had moved to the cities, he made a simple but profound observation: the average daily stool weight of the hunter-gatherers was 2 pounds (900 g); of the city dwellers, only 4 ounces (115 g). The hunter-gatherers had none of our modern chronic diseases, while their cousins had them all. The difference? Fiber. And fiber is food for good gut bacteria. Hunter-gatherers ate an average of 100 to 150 grams a day. Our modern Western diet contains only 8 to 15 grams a day, and fewer than 5 percent of Americans consume the recommended daily amount (about 30 grams a day).[21] The concept of the microbiome was not even on the radar, but the link between diet, stool, and chronic disease was obvious long ago.

In Burkitt's words, "In Africa, treating people who live largely off the land on vegetables they grow, I hardly ever saw cases of many of the most common diseases in the United States and England—including coronary heart disease, adult-onset diabetes, varicose veins, obesity, diverticulitis, appendicitis, gallstones, dental cavities, hemorrhoids, hiatal hernias, and constipation. Western diets are so low on bulk and so dense in calories, that our intestines just don't pass enough volume to remain healthy."[22]

Élie Metchnikoff, who won the Nobel Prize in 1908 for his work in immunology, first noticed the link between gut microbes, health, and longevity by studying centenarians in the Balkans who ate yogurt.[23] He posited the link between gut bacteria leaking across the intestinal lining and inflammation and chronic disease, especially heart disease. His theories initially took hold but were then dismissed by conventional medicine. Now the microbiome is the subject of intense research in the private and public sector, including in the NIH's Human Microbiome Project. Today, probiotics are a multibillion-dollar industry. Metchnikoff's prescient work laid the foundation for the microbiome revolution and even fecal microbiota transplantation (FMT).

The gut ecosystem, long ignored by medicine, is now identified to be linked to nearly all chronic disease, including cancer, heart disease, obesity, type 2 diabetes, Parkinson's, and dementia, as well as to autoimmune disease, allergies, mood disorders, and even autism.

So, what's up with poop? Your gut contains as many bacterial cells as your body has human cells, but there are more than 1,000 species of bacteria containing a hundred times as much DNA as your own DNA. In other words, you are only 1 percent human! It is estimated that in an average human blood sample, a third to a half of the metabolites are from gut bacteria. Good bugs create health. Bad bugs create disease.[24] It's impossible to achieve optimal health and longevity with an out-of-balance gut.

The state of modern poop is frighteningly dangerous. If we examine the feces of hunter-gatherers, it comprises vastly different microbes than that of modern-day humans. Why has modern poop become a cesspool rather than a compost pile? We live in a gut-busting world. The combination of our Western diet—low in fiber, high in processed foods, sugar, food additives, pesticides, and herbicides (especially the microbiome-destroying weed killer glyphosate, used on 70 percent of global crops)—and gut-busting drugs such as acid blockers, anti-inflammatories (like ibuprofen or aspirin), and antibiotics has radically changed the makeup of our microbiome, fostering *dysbiosis,* imbalance of gut bacteria, rather than symbiosis. The result is a toxic microbiome, a disease-causing, age-accelerating mess.

Fun fact: 25 percent of calories from breast milk, in the form of special sugars called oligosaccharides, are not digestible by babies.[25] Why are these special sugars there? To feed the infant's microbiome, especially *Bifidobacterium infantis,* the microbe responsible for the development of a healthy immune system. Their absence is linked to colic, allergies, asthma, eczema, and autoimmunity in addition to generalized inflammation. There is even a name for this condition: *newborn gut deficiency.* A common antibiotic given to the mother days before labor and delivery will wipe out this keystone species, so even a vaginal delivery won't protect the baby.[26] Thankfully one company has created a highly researched supplement probiotic called Evivo, containing a specialized strain of *B. infantis,* that can be given to babies at birth. It will colonize in their gut and avert the dangers of its absence.

How does an unhealthy gut lead to chronic disease and accelerated aging and what can we do about it?[27] While the research is growing exponentially and there is much to learn, we know a lot already. Bad bugs grow like weeds because we constantly fertilize them with sugar, flour, and processed foods, and we under-fertilize the good bugs with fiber and polyphenols. These bad bugs can cause an increase in intestinal permeability, otherwise known as *leaky gut.*

Your gut is a long tube that goes from mouth to anus. It is essentially a closed system full of foreign things—food and bugs. Food is broken down by a healthy gut to its component parts—amino acids, fatty acids, sugars. These are absorbed through the intestinal cells held together tightly in a single layer by connectors called *tight junctions*. Right under the one-cell layer separating you from a sewer is about 70 percent of your immune system. Why is it there? The gut is where you encounter the most foreign antigens that you need to defend against.

When that barrier is damaged, undigested food proteins and bacterial toxins and proteins "leak" in between the cells, and your immune system does exactly what it is supposed to do: create an immune response, driving up inflammation throughout the body, accelerating most disease and aging itself.

Billions of dollars are pouring into microbiome research. Many companies now offer microbiome and stool testing. Others are bringing to market new probiotics and prebiotics and even fecal transplant pills (yes, poop pills). Much work is yet to be done. However, the foundational principles of microbiome restoration have long been used in functional medicine to restore a healthy gut microbiome, and they are a key part of the Young Forever Program outlined in Part III.

HALLMARK 9: STEM CELL EXHAUSTION—THE DECLINE OF OUR BODY'S REJUVENATION SYSTEM

We are all familiar with how stem cells work, even if we don't realize it. How does your skin heal after a cut? Stem cells are recruited and secrete healing and growth factors that trigger your body into repair and renewal. It's miraculous. Starfish and salamanders can grow new limbs. Even our own livers can grow back after 90 percent has been removed.

That single cell from which we started is called an *embryonic stem cell*. It holds within it your entire genome. Everywhere in our tissues, we have and produce adult stem cells called *mesenchymal stem cells* (MSCs). The adult stem cells in the bone marrow that make your red and white blood cells and platelets are called *hematopoietic stem cells* (HSCs). But as we age, our stem cells age too. They become less able to repair and renew our cells, tissues, and organs.

As with all other hallmarks of aging, decline in our stem cell function is caused in large part by our exposome—our diet, exercise, sleep, stress, environmental toxins, allergens, and microbes, all things we have control over. Exciting innovations in regenerative medicine—including stem cell therapy and plasma rejuvenation, which I cover in Chapter 11—can help us address the aging of our stem cells. But with the right exposome modifications available to us all, they may not even be necessary.

HALLMARK 10: INFLAMMAGING—THE FIRE THAT DRIVES CHRONIC DISEASE AND SHORTENS LIFE

All the other hallmarks play a role in this final hallmark of aging: a dysfunction in immune functioning called *inflammaging*.[28] Two seemingly contradictory things happen as we age. First, our immune system itself ages and our ability to fight infections and cancer declines. This is called *immunosenescence*. That's why the risk of dying from infections and from cancer both increase dramatically as we get older. While our immune system's ability to seek out and kill infections and remove cancer cells declines, other parts of the immune system are activated, driving *sterile inflammation,* inflammation caused by things other than infections, like tissue damage, toxins, antigens, and others. COVID-19 has made us aware of something called the *cytokine storm,* a type of inflammation that causes an overwhelming flood of inflammatory messengers that can ultimately kill us. Consider abnormal aging a slow, smoldering sterile cytokine storm.

As we've discussed, cytokines are molecules produced by our immune system to fight infection and cancer. When dysregulated, though, they cause our immune system to overheat, resulting in allergy and autoimmunity. Why do we lose our ability to fight infections and cancer while at the same time finding ourselves in a sea of cytokines? Every age-related chronic disease is both caused by and causes inflammation in a self-perpetuating cycle.

Why does this happen? In our evolutionary past survival depended on our immune system's ability to fight infection and kill cancer cells when we were young. This was less important as our reproductive period waned. Keeping us free from infection and cancer doesn't matter as much if we can't have more babies. The thymus, the seat of our immune system, shrinks and nearly disappears as we age. The insults that accompany life—poor diet, stress, inactivity, poor sleep, environmental toxins, changes to our microbiome, social isolation—all drive inflammation, but not inflammation that is directed at cancer cells or infections. This paradoxical phenomenon of a strong immune system when we are young and a weak one when we are old is called *antagonistic pleiotropy,* which simply means that what worked for us when we were young becomes problematic as we age, a trade-off between reproduction and longevity.

As a functional medicine doctor, I often think of myself as an *inflammologist.* The key is not to shut down the inflammation or the inflammatory response but to balance inflammation (*some* inflammation is a good thing!) by removing the root causes. The primary driver is our modern diet. It is pro-inflammatory, high in sugar and starch, low in fiber, awash in refined oils, nutrient poor, and phytonutrient depleted. In other words, a perfect recipe for disease, inflammation, and aging. This diet also harms our microbiome, causing an overgrowth of inflammatory bugs and depletion of anti-inflammatory bugs, driving leaky gut. Since most of our immune system is in the gut, this is a big contributor to inflammation. Add to that the load of 84,000 environmental chemicals (fewer than 1 percent of which have been tested for safety)[29] in our food, water, air, and household cleaning and personal care products, and our exposure to mercury in fish and dental fillings, lead in the environment from leaded gas (still in our soil) and leaded paint, heavy metals and particulate pollution from coal-burning plants, and arsenic in food and water, and we have a perfect storm for inflammation. Even psychological stress and lack of sleep, a product of our overworked, under-loved culture, drives inflammation.

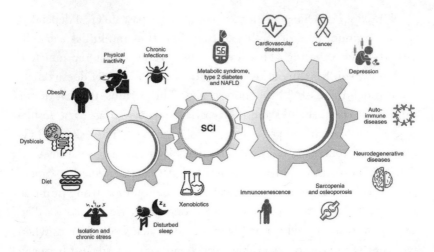

Source: Furman D, Campisi J, Verdin E, et al. "Chronic Inflammation in the Etiology of Disease across the Life Span." *Nat Med.* 2019;25(12):1822–32. Note: SCI: systemic chronic inflammation. Illustration courtesy of Dr David Furman.

All the hallmarks of aging result in even more inflammation—worsening DNA damage, mitochondrial injury, free-radical accumulation, altered nutrient signaling, not enough autophagy and cellular cleanup, too many zombie cells, damaged proteins, and epigenetic changes. Together, these changes lead to a flood of cytokines that damage and prematurely age the body.

The good news is that limiting inflammation and activating our anti-inflammatory pathways is not hard to do. The Young Forever Program maps out how to boost our ability to fight infection and cancer while reducing the process of *inflammaging*. How can we do that? By following an anti-inflammatory diet, activating the longevity switches with time-restricted eating and phytochemicals, using *hormesis* (see Chapter 10) to activate our body's innate healing systems, exercising, reducing stress, getting good sleep, avoiding and eliminating environmental toxins, and optimizing the microbiome. Key phytochemicals and supplements, and novel therapies—including stem cell therapy, exosomes, plasma exchange, and other treatments—may all be part of an anti-inflammatory, health-creating, life-extending strategy.

The Young Forever Program is designed to address the hallmarks and imbalances that drive disease and aging.

Cutting-edge research has given us a window into the profound mysteries and complexities of our bodies. Einstein said, "I don't want to know the spectrum of this or that element. I want to know the thoughts of God. The rest are details." We are at a moment in science where the thoughts of God are being revealed, just as they were in the discovery of the laws of physics. Physics has very few laws that explain nearly all observed phenomena. The laws of biology are now emerging.

Pierre Laplace, the eighteenth-century physicist, said, "The simplicity of nature is not to be measured by that of our conceptions. Infinitely varied in its effects, nature is simple only in its causes, and its economy consists in producing a great number of phenomena, often very complicated, by means of a small number of general laws." The hallmarks are part of the newly discovered laws of biology, a few things that go wrong and that can explain a myriad of disease and aging itself.

Now that we know the hallmarks of aging, we can focus on their underlying causes—the imbalances in our basic biological networks mapped out by functional medicine that result in chronic disease, premature aging, pain, and frailty. Once we understand the root causes of the hallmarks of aging, we are poised to go beyond just prevention or treatment and into an era of rejuvenation, regeneration, radical health optimization, health span improvement, and life span extension.

Chapter 5

Dying of Too Much or Too Little: Why Balance Matters

Those who disobey the laws of Heaven and Earth have a lifetime of calamities, while those who follow the laws remain free from dangerous illness.

—HUANGDI NEIJING (THE YELLOW EMPEROR'S CLASSIC OF INTERNAL MEDICINE)

How many chemical reactions happen every second in the human body? A million? A trillion? Nope. Thirty-seven billion billion. That's twenty-seven zeros! It is beyond our minds' ability to comprehend the complexities of the human organism. This magical dance of molecules and chemical reactions underlies all health, disease, and aging. Learning how to fine-tune these reactions, to facilitate healing, repair, and regeneration, is at the heart of functional medicine.

The hallmarks of aging are *how* our biology becomes out of balance. Conventional medicine describes the *what:* what disease, what pathway is dysfunctional, what drug to take. The model of functional medicine guides us to the *why,* to the root causes of diseases and aging. Many longevity research efforts focus on just treating the hallmarks of aging, without treating their underlying causes. That's where functional medicine comes in. What causes the hallmarks in the first place? Imbalance—too much bad stuff, not enough good stuff.

The beauty of the human organism is that we don't have to know its every gene, protein, metabolite, or microbe. We simply need to know what creates imbalance or balance, and thankfully it is not millions of things. It is a few simple things.

In functional medicine, we ask just two questions to figure out what's causing dysfunction in the body's ecosystem. First, what do you need to get rid of that is causing the imbalance? Second, what do you need to put into the system to help restore balance? In other words, how is your exposome harming or helping your body?

While genes play a role in our health, our disease risks, and our potential for longevity, they play far less of a role than we had imagined. The exposome determines 90 percent of our disease and aging risk. Our genes and every aspect of our biology respond in real time to our exposome. While some populations, like those in the Blue Zones, experience great longevity, when they adopt a modern diet and lifestyle, their disease risks go up and their longevity plummets. While the various Blue Zones are located across the world, they all are in places where the good stuff, like whole foods, movement, and community, is abundant and the bad stuff, like processed food, a sedentary lifestyle, chronic stress, and environmental toxins, is mostly absent. That's good news for all of us because it means we have tremendous power over our health and life span.

Evolution set up our biology to function in very particular ways. The fact that 93 percent of Americans are metabolically unhealthy and suffering from some degree of pre-diabetes or type 2 diabetes (which is at the root of rapid aging and heart disease, cancer, and dementia) is largely due to the burden of too many things we never evolved to handle and not enough of the things designed to help us thrive.[1]

What do we need to reduce or eliminate to create health?

- Our modern ultraprocessed diet,[2] loaded with sugar and flour[3] as well as hydrogenated oils and too many refined oils
- Environmental toxins (84,000 new compounds just since 1900)
- Certain types of infections (latent viruses, bacteria, and tick-borne illness) and microbiome imbalances

- Gut-damaging medication, including antibiotics, anti-inflammatories, and acid blockers
- Allergens and food sensitivities
- Inactivity
- Chronic stressors of modern life (physical and psychological)
- Social isolation and loneliness

What do we need to increase or add to create health? What are the ingredients for health?

- Whole, real, unprocessed foods
- Wild regeneratively-raised or grass- or pasture-raised meats and eggs and fatty fish
- Fiber
- Phytonutrients
- Micronutrients (e.g., vitamin D, zinc, magnesium, B vitamins, omega-3 fatty acids)
- Optimal hormone levels (supported by healthy lifestyle or bioidentical hormone replacement)
- Adequate and ideal light exposure at the right times of day
- Optimal hydration
- Clean air
- Exercise and movement
- Restorative practices (yoga, meditation, breath work)
- Sleep and healthy circadian rhythms
- Community, love, and belonging
- Meaning and purpose

By adding the good stuff and removing the bad, you activate your body's natural healing systems, its innate intelligence that is designed to create health. We have far more control over our biology than most of us have ever imagined. While it is impossible to optimize for all the good stuff or eliminate all the bad stuff all the time, it is important to build a lifestyle that automatically makes all of it just a little simpler and habitual. That is what the Young Forever Program is designed to help you do.

So, what causes our biology to become unbalanced and drives the hallmarks of aging?

OUR INFLAMMATORY AND AGING-PROMOTING DIET

The most important regulator of disease is our diet. Food is medicine. But it can also be poison. Today's Western processed-food diet accounts, conservatively, for 11 million deaths globally a year,[4] likely a gross underestimate considering that 41 million people a year die from a chronic disease—this is 71 percent of all deaths worldwide.[5] Tobacco use accounts for 7 million of those deaths. Environmental toxins, often called *autogens* (creating autoimmune disease) and *obesogens,* contribute synergistically with poor diet to promote the hallmarks of aging and account for 9 million additional deaths a year. Diet plays a significant role in heart disease, cancer, diabetes, and dementia. These diseases were rare or absent just 150 years ago. Hospital records from the early 1800s clearly demonstrate the rarity of type 2 diabetes and heart disease and show that they are not inevitable consequences of being human, but adaptations to a bad set of circumstances.[6]

The United States has created the worst diet in the world and exported it to nearly every country on the planet, which is why 31 million of those global deaths from chronic disease are in low- or middle-income countries, double the deaths from infectious disease.

The flood of industrialized food into the marketplace has caused inexorable harm to humanity and the planet. In my book *Food Fix: How to Save Our Health, Our Economy, Our Communities, and Our Planet— One Bite at a Time,* I explore in detail the harms and solutions. Today, 60 percent of our diet is ultraprocessed food. For every 10 percent of your diet that is ultraprocessed food, your risk of death goes up by 14 percent.[7] You do the math. It's not a pretty picture. And for kids it is worse—67 percent of their diet is ultraprocessed food.[8] The unbelievable load of sugar and flour, 152 pounds (69 kg) and 133 pounds (60 kg) per person per year, respectively, is deadly. Add to that a thousandfold increase in processed and refined oils since 1900, 5 pounds (2.2 kg) of food additives and preservatives consumed annually by the average American, and the fact that 90 percent of Americans don't consume the minimum recommended amounts of protective foods such as fruits and vegetables, and you have a perfect storm for exacerbating all the hallmarks of aging.[9] Hyperpalatable, ultraprocessed food also triggers overeating (about 500 extra calories a day for those who eat those foods), flooding and harming our nutrient-sensing pathways that regulate autophagy, inflammation, and DNA repair, and causing mitochondrial injury and damage to proteins. These damaged proteins trigger further inflammation in a destructive cycle of inflammaging.[10]

Our diet drives harmful changes in our microbiome, causing leaky gut, and changes to our immune system, causing low-grade *metabolic endotoxemia,* a fancy way of saying that our crappy diet leads to obesity by fertilizing bad toxin-releasing, inflammation-causing bacteria. Also when we overprocess or fry food, it increases oxidation and the production of free radicals, further driving inflammation. And of course, the sugar and refined grains that make up the bulk of our diet cause more oxidative stress and more inflammation.

It's not only what we get too much of, but what we are lacking. The lack of immune-modulating, anti-inflammatory micronutrients, including vitamin D, zinc, magnesium, and omega-3 fats, drives even more inflammation. Omega-3 fats and their protective components, including *resolvins*[11] (compounds that put the brakes on inflammation), help lower overall inflammation. High intakes of refined omega-6 oils and low intakes of wild foods and fatty fish high in omega-3 fats promote more inflammation. The mountains of added salt in processed foods and lack of potassium (from fruits and vegetables) in our diets worsen inflammation.[12] All in all, if we were to design the perfect diet to create an epidemic of chronic disease and a shortened life span, it would be our current industrialized, toxic diet.

OUR SEDENTARY DISEASE-PROMOTING LIFESTYLE

Our exposome encompasses not only our diet but also our patterns of exercise, stress, sleep, circadian rhythm, nighttime light exposure, and social isolation. There is a great evolutionary mismatch between our current lifestyle and environment and our genes and biology. Our ancient world was one of few environmental toxins except for the odd poisonous mushroom, of synchronizing our biological rhythms to the sun and moon and no artificial light, of no chronic stressors, of 8 or 9 hours of sleep a night, of regular and significant physical activity, of close-knit tribal communities and family systems.[13] In short, a world dramatically different from the one we find ourselves in today. This deviation from the automatic inputs of whole foods, movement, sleep, natural light,[14] and clean air and water has driven the cascade of biological dysfunction in our billions of chemical reactions, resulting in the hallmarks of aging that drive disease and death.[15] Our ancestors were constantly on the move—foraging for food, hunting, avoiding predators, and seeking shelter. They were not sitting behind desks, cruising in their cars, binge-watching Netflix, or doomscrolling. The lack of natural movement today is a harmful mismatch with our biology.

Without having to go to the gym or get a trainer or buy running shoes, our ancestors moved, and they moved a lot, using their bodies as designed. Only 23 percent of Americans get the recommended amount of daily physical activity.[16] And half of us are completely physically inactive. That's deadly for us. When we don't move our bodies, push our hearts to pump, or strengthen our muscles, not only do we become soft and doughy but our muscles become fountains of inflammation, altered hormones, and disease due to sarcopenia. We become more insulin resistant, our blood pressure goes up, our stress hormones increase while our sex hormones decrease, our bones waste away, and our risk of heart disease, cancer, diabetes, fatty liver, and dementia all go way up. Not exercising results in more belly or visceral fat, which is

almost literally a fire in the belly, spewing forth cytokines that accelerate a cascade of hormonal and metabolic destruction that promotes
weight gain, even more belly fat, and inflammaging. In fact, shatter-
ing the old idea that weight gain is the result of eating too much and
not exercising enough (eating more calories than we burn), science
proves that it is the slow accumulation of belly fat from eating too
much of the wrong thing that makes us overeat more and exercise
less.[17] Belly fat is "hungry fat." It slows our metabolism and fat burning,
makes us hungry, and turns us into couch potatoes.

Lack of exercise accelerates all the hallmarks of aging: mitochondrial dysfunction, the nutrient-sensing pathways, inflammaging, abnormal proteins, DNA damage, telomere shortening, zombie cells,
epigenetic changes, and stem cell exhaustion. Exercise is one simple
intervention that can help reverse most of the hallmarks of aging.[18]

If exercise could be put in a pill, it might be the most powerful
health-promoting longevity strategy ever. Simply walking for 20 minutes a day can cut your risks of heart disease, diabetes, cancer, and
dementia by 40 percent.[19] In fact, one of the best predictors of life
expectancy is your fitness level measured by something called VO_2
max, an indirect measurement of the efficiency of your metabolism
and fitness level.[20] The fitter you are, the healthier and longer you live.
Time to get moving! However, despite how critical exercise is to our
health and longevity, you cannot exercise your way out of a bad diet.[21]

SOCIAL DISEASES: OUR SOCIAL ENVIRONMENT AND HEALTH

In the immediate aftermath of the 2010 earthquake in Haiti, I gathered a medical team and was among the first to arrive to help at the
general hospital in Port-au-Prince, the epicenter of the disaster. We
brought with us the late Paul Farmer from Partners in Health, who
had helped cure multidrug-resistant tuberculosis and AIDS in the
poorest country in the Western Hemisphere, a population that had
been abandoned by the global public health community as too poor
and difficult to treat. He did it not with better drugs, but with the

power of *accompaniment,* a model that engaged neighbors to help neighbors. People accompanied each other to health. They were trained as community health workers. Dr Farmer talked about the roots of illness as social, or what he called *structural violence,* the social, economic, and political conditions that drive disease. Today we refer to these as *social determinants of health.* The language matters less than the science, which clearly shows the impact of social stressors on our health. We know that loneliness is one of the biggest risk factors for disease and that feeling powerless is as big a risk factor as smoking or poor diet.[22] It became clear to me that most chronic diseases are not "noncommunicable" but highly contagious. That our social connections impact our health. You are 171 percent more likely to be obese if your friends are, but only 40 percent more likely if your siblings are, and obesity significantly shortens your life.[23] An obese child ends up living 13 fewer years than a normal-weight child. Now 40 percent of our kids are overweight.

Today we have moved so far from our evolutionary tribal cultures, or even from the richness of our family and social systems of a hundred years ago. My mother grew up in the 1930s in Brooklyn with all of her grandparents, uncles, aunts, and cousins living on the same block. Now I don't know any of my cousins except two or three (out of hundreds in my extended family). The Blue Zones are renowned not only for their whole foods diet and built-in exercise but also for their tightly knit fabric of social connections, like the *moai,* a small group created at birth within which Okinawans live, play, and die.

Chronic stress from social isolation translates into biological signals that accelerate the hallmarks of aging, including inflammation, mitochondrial dysfunction, epigenetic damage, telomere shortening, and altered nutrient sensing.[24] There is now a whole new scientific field called psycho-neuro-endo-immunology that studies the way stress makes you sick and age faster. Your genes, immune system, microbiome, hormones, and more are listening to and taking instruction from your thoughts and feelings and beliefs. Addressing your stress levels is key to healthy aging.

Building community, creating belonging, nurturing relationships and support groups, even being in a knitting or bowling group is associated with better health and longevity. In 2011, Pastor Rick Warren, Dr Daniel Amen, and I created a faith-based wellness program, the Daniel Plan, founded on the principle that getting healthy is a team sport. Small, self-directed support groups in Saddleback Church were taught about healthy living. In one year, 15,000 people lost 250,000 pounds (113,000 kg) and transformed their health using the power of community as medicine.

Biological aging can result from psychological, social, or physical stressors—from lack of sleep or lack of physical touch. A new area of research called *sociogenomics* explains how our social and psychological environments influence our gene expression.[25] This is not an abstract notion or theory. Our thoughts, our beliefs, our relationships or lack thereof, all drive measurable changes in gene expression, affecting genes that control inflammation and our stress hormones. Loss of a sense of agency, rejection, loneliness, social isolation, and trauma impact our immune system, our hormones, and our gut.[26]

While trauma that occurs at any stage in life can have negative impacts on our health, early childhood trauma leaves us more vulnerable to disease and death. A high score on the ACE (Adverse Childhood Experiences) Questionnaire is highly correlated with mortality.[27] But our environment is not necessarily the only problem; it is the story we make from it. Dr Gabor Maté, a leading expert in the impact of trauma on our physical and mental health, suggests that trauma is not what happens to us, but the meaning we make from what happens to us. Healing from trauma can be extremely difficult, and I recommend working with a trained therapist for the best support, but it's also extremely important, for both your short-term and long-term health. In Part III I will explore promising emerging trauma therapies including ketamine-, MDMA-, and psilocybin-assisted therapy.

Our social determinants of health, including community, relationships, stress, trauma, and sense of purpose and belonging, are just as important for our health as what we eat and how we move. If you're feeling lonely, stressed, isolated, or powerless, your biology, your cells, your microbiome, literally "hear" your thoughts and feelings, driving inflammation and disease. Working with a trained professional to heal from trauma, serious life events, or struggles like chronic depression is important, but there are simple daily practices that help improve your social and emotional well-being, including practicing gratitude, prioritizing self-care, being of service to others, joining a community, and starting meditation. Whatever strategy you develop for health and longevity, it must include nurturing and developing your own social fabric of belonging, meaning, and purpose.

THE HARM OF INADEQUATE SLEEP

It may surprise you to hear that one of the major physical stresses on us modern humans is driven by the discovery of electricity. The light bulb, however useful, may be responsible for more deaths than we can imagine. The disruption of our circadian rhythms with nighttime light, and now with increasing screen use, has shortened our evolutionary sleep patterns by 2 hours. This is more harmful than most of us realize. It has raised the risk of insulin resistance, obesity, type 2 diabetes, heart disease, and death from all causes.[28] Lack of sleep drives most of the hallmarks of aging, especially inflammation,[29] mitochondrial damage, and altered hormonal and nutrient-sensing pathways.[30] It triggers changes that make you crave sugar and carbs and prevents your body from healing, repair, and rejuvenation. The brain, for example, has its own detoxification system, the *glymphatic system,* which cleans up all the metabolic waste and garbage that accumulates during the day. Lack of sleep impairs that system, increasing the risk for depression, dementia, and more.

Our daily biological rhythms are controlled in part by our exposure to light: sunlight in the morning and darkness at night. Exposure to blue-spectrum light at atypical biologic times (like before bed) increases alertness and arousal, alters our circadian rhythm, drives inflammation, and impairs our mitochondrial function.[31] Even if you get enough sleep, it can still be harmful. Shift work is known to increase the risk of obesity, heart disease, and cancer and cause early death. "Let there be light" should be qualified as "Let there be light *during the day*"! Thankfully there are ways to reduce blue-light exposure at night with blue-blocker glasses; screen settings on phones, tablets, and computers; and special light bulbs that remove blue-spectrum light.

When you learn how to reset sleep and circadian rhythms, you pull powerful levers for longevity.

TROUBLE WITH MICROBES: BAD BUGS, INFLAMMATION, AND OBESITY

Something rotten inside us causes us to get sick and age prematurely. Age-related changes in our gut, the result of a lifetime of gut-unfriendly habits, trigger inflammation, insulin resistance, and obesity, worsening all the hallmarks of aging.[32] Paleo poop was quite different from modern poop. Happy gut bugs kept immune systems well regulated and free of allergies, autoimmunity, heart disease, cancer, diabetes, and obesity. Our ancestors didn't live a hypersterilized life. Living and playing in the dirt were the norm. Changes in our diet, overuse of antibiotics, acid-blocking drugs, and anti-inflammatory drugs, and high rates of unnecessary C-sections have created a perfect storm for *dysbiosis*,[33] a toxic imbalance of bad gut bugs. In Moises Velasquez-Manoff's *An Epidemic of Absence* and Martin J. Blaser's *Missing Microbes,* the health and longevity consequences of this change in our microbiome are vividly mapped out.[34]

Too much bad bacteria leads to high levels of a molecule called *zonulin* that loosens the tight junctions in your intestinal barrier and increases leaky gut. Zonulin is found in obese adults and children[35] and people with type 2 diabetes, fatty liver, heart disease, infertility, autoimmune disease, and cancer. It predicts systemic inflammation and frailty.[36] Zonulin was first discovered by Dr Alessio Fasano while he was studying cholera. Cholera and other toxic bacteria trigger zonulin release. But it is not only bad bugs that trigger zonulin. Gluten is the biggest zonulin-triggering culprit today. And our modern dwarf wheat has way more gliadin (or gluten proteins) than our ancient wheat.[37] This may explain the 400 percent increase in celiac disease in the last 50 years and the dramatic rise in non–celiac gluten sensitivity. Gluten is a huge trigger of inflammation, gut damage, autoimmunity, heart disease, cancer, dementia, and aging itself.

The exploding field of microbiome research is already providing us with novel ways to reset our gut, including prebiotics, probiotics, post-biotics, symbiotics, polyphenol blends, and even fecal transplants to reestablish a healthy microbial ecosystem. It's hard to believe, but in the not-too-distant future we may be swallowing frozen poop pills from healthy donors to reboot our gut. Early studies show that fecal microbiota transplantation can reverse obesity, type 2 diabetes, autism, autoimmune diseases, and more.

As we've discussed, infections also drive inflammation as we age. *Immunosenescence,* the aging of our immune system, impairs our ability to manage all the pathogens that we easily manage when we are young. For example, a case of chicken pox as a child will make you a little sick, but it then goes dormant for decades until a stressor triggers its reactivation as shingles when you are older. Many viruses such as cytomegalovirus, Epstein-Barr, hepatitis C, and other infectious agents have been linked to accelerated aging.[38] Our modern inflammatory, immune-disrupting lifestyle may predispose us to the bad effects of all the viruses and parasites our ancestors lived with and managed quite well.[39] New infections, including tick-borne infections such as Lyme disease, COVID-19, and long COVID syndrome, have introduced something new to the mix. These are persistent, often debilitating infections that are hard to treat and create systemic inflammation. We have a lot to learn about how we can best live in harmony with our little creatures and not let them aggravate our immune systems and accelerate aging.

The Young Forever Program provides a road map for optimizing gut healing in service of preventing disease and enhancing your quality and length of life.

THE TOXIC TIDE OF CHEMICALS AND METALS

Two things we learn little to nothing about in medical school are nutrition and the role of toxins in human health (aside from acute poisoning). Over the last 200 years an unprecedented rise in exposure to petrochemical compounds and heavy metals has contributed to our chronic disease burden and accelerated aging, acting through many of the pathways outlined in Chapter 4, on the hallmarks of aging. Environmental toxins are increasingly recognized as significant contributors to chronic disease, including heart disease, diabetes, obesity, cancer, hormonal diseases such as infertility and low sperm counts, autoimmunity, neurodegenerative disease, autism, and more.

More than 84,000 new chemicals have been introduced into commercial products and have found their way into our water, air, and food since 1900, including pesticides, herbicides, plastics, flame retardants, phthalates, per- and polyfluoroalkyl substances, bisphenols, polycyclic aromatic hydrocarbons, and heavy metals including arsenic, lead, and mercury—to name just a few.[40] These are found in home-cleaning and personal-care products, prescription medications, lawn-care products, and more. Most of these compounds have not been adequately tested on humans, and if they have, it has been as isolated compounds in small amounts without considering the synergistic nature of multiple exposures. Biopsies of human fat reveal that each of us is a toxic waste dump full of even banned compounds such as DDT, PCBs, and dioxin. The average newborn has 287 known toxins in their umbilical cord blood even before they take their first breath.[41] If we were food, we wouldn't be safe to eat.

Toxins wreak havoc through multiple pathways. Some have been called *obesogens* for their impact on our metabolism and insulin resistance and are known causes of obesity, type 2 diabetes, and heart disease. Some are also considered *autogens* for their impact on autoimmune diseases and their ability to drive inflammation throughout our body. Some are known as endocrine disruptors, or *xenobiotics,* causing hormonal chaos in our sex and thyroid hormones. And, of course, many are carcinogens. How do these compounds cause havoc on our health and accelerate disease and aging? They drive changes and injury in all our biological networks—our gut, immune system, energy production, detoxification system, lymph and circulatory systems, hormones and neurotransmitters, and even our cell structures by directly damaging cells and cellular components. Toxins damage our DNA and our mitochondria, interfere with our nutrient-sensing pathways, shorten our telomeres, alter our proteins and their function, cause cells to age, exhaust our stem cells, and adversely impact our epigenome. They even damage our microbiome and cause leaky gut.

Reducing exposures and optimizing your detoxification systems, processes outlined in the Young Forever Program, are critical to preventing, treating, and reversing chronic disease and aiding longevity.

OPTIMIZING THE INGREDIENTS FOR HEALTH AND LONGEVITY: DYING OF TOO LITTLE

One of the central tenets of functional medicine is this: We are sick because of either too much of something that is hurting us or not enough of the good stuff needed to help us thrive and function optimally. Think of these as the ingredients for health. Like it or not, we are biological organisms and must follow the laws of nature. If we are growing a beautiful garden, we know we must prepare the soil and add compost, nutrients, water, sunlight, and the right temperature. With too little of these necessary ingredients, our garden won't thrive. Our bodies are the same. Thankfully the list of what our human garden needs is relatively short, and focusing on putting the highest-quality "ingredients" for health into our bodies to bring us health and longevity is relatively simple.

What are these "ingredients" for health? The obvious ones. Nutrient-dense real food; optimal levels of nutrients, vitamins, minerals, and phytonutrients; the right balance of hormones; the right types of exercise; optimal quality and duration of sleep; deep, restorative practices like meditation or breath work; the right light at the right times, honoring our circadian rhythms; clean water and air; the right mind-set and mastering our mind's negative inner dialogue, which registers in every cell in our body; meaning and purpose; community and con-nection and love. These are the fundamental building blocks of human health, most of which we as a culture do not prioritize.

Functional medicine is a system of thinking that allows us to diag-nose and treat the excesses and deficiencies to optimize every one of our biological networks. So, let's turn to Part II, where we'll explore how everything in the Young Forever Program works to balance and opti-mize your seven core biological systems. Using this road map, we will then dive into foundational practices for optimizing your diet, exercise, stress management, sleep, and social well-being. Next, we'll explore the powerful science and practice of *hormesis,* the little stresses that help you heal disease, maximize your health, and activate your longevity path-ways. Finally, we'll survey more advanced innovations available now and coming soon that hold the promise to supercharge your health, reverse aging, and extend your years of vibrant, healthy life.

PART II

OPTIMIZING YOUR HEALTH SPAN AND LIFE SPAN

Chapter 6

Foundations of Longevity: Balancing Your Seven Core Biological Systems

Nothing in science—nothing in life for that matter—makes sense without theory. It is our nature to put all knowledge into context in order to tell a story and to re-create the world by this means.

—E. O. WILSON

Many of the hallmarks of aging identified by longevity researchers— such as mitochondrial dysfunction, imbalances in the microbiome, inflammation, dysfunction in nutrient sensing, and the hormonal changes that occur with aging—are, in fact, describing the fundamental biological networks of functional medicine that must be cared for and optimized to avoid disease and create longevity. This new theory of health, disease, and aging is a profound paradigm shift.

Let's briefly review the seven core networks that underlie disease and aging, networks that must be in balance for us to be healthy, including your microbiome, immune system, mitochondria, detoxification, circulation and transportation, communication, and structural system.

CORE SYSTEM 1: ASSIMILATING NUTRIENTS, DIGESTION, AND THE MICROBIOME

Medicine has long held a two-dimensional view of the gut. It is simply a tube from mouth to anus designed to absorb nutrients and fluids.

Other than major gut diseases like reflux, irritable bowel, and inflammatory bowel diseases, doctors mostly considered the gut to be irrelevant when it came to understanding our overall health. But the gut, it turns out, is at the center of our health.

In Chapter 4, on the hallmarks of aging, you learned how the microbiome plays a critical role in our health and longevity and what causes it to become out of balance. A recent study found that transplanting stool from a young mouse to an old mouse made the old mouse young;[1] the stool transplant reduced inflammation through the system including the brain, eye, and gut. Similarly, they found that putting old poop into young mice made the young mice older, increasing brain, eye, and gut inflammation and causing a leaky gut. While we may not quite be at the stage of harvesting youthful poop to transplant into aging humans, we are not that far off. This just underscores the critical importance of understanding how to tend your inner garden throughout your life and healing the gut as a core strategy for reversing disease and extending life span.

Your gut may be the most important and complex system in your body. It must break down and digest food into its component parts—amino acids, sugars and fats, fiber, vitamins, minerals, phytonutrients—and assimilate these life-giving compounds while keeping out harmful microbes and partially digested food particles that contribute to most diseases. To be healthy, your microbiome must also be healthy, comprised of optimal levels of healthy bacteria that optimize the gut ecosystem and provide important beneficial metabolites we absorb and use to regulate our health. It must not have too many nasty bugs, which cause inflammation, and toxic metabolites, which are absorbed, can disturb every aspect of our health, and have been implicated in nearly every chronic disease.[2]

Learning to tend your inner garden is essential to health and longevity. You feed your garden every day. With every bite of food, you feed the good bugs or the bad bugs, and you heal the lining of the gut or damage it. Damage to the gut lining, or leaky gut, is one of the most important factors driving inflammation and adversely affecting nearly all the hallmarks of aging. The key to a healthy gut is a whole foods diet high in prebiotic (fiber) and probiotic foods and abundant in phytochemicals from colorful plant foods. The discovery that our good microbes love phytochemicals such as polyphenols contained within colorful vegetables and fruit gives us a powerful way to feed the gut.

The Young Forever Program will help you identify and fix the imbalances in your gut.

CORE SYSTEM 2: DEFENSE AND REPAIR—OUR IMMUNE AND INFLAMMATORY SYSTEM

The body has only so many ways of saying "ouch," but many things can hurt it. And infectious disease doesn't affect everyone the same way, as we have seen with COVID-19. Those who are pre-inflamed because of obesity, type 2 diabetes, heart disease, and inflammaging are at a dramatically higher risk of severe disease, hospitalization, and death from COVID-19. Same virus, very different outcomes. Many insults that modern humans experience lead to the final common pathway of inflammation: toxins, allergens, microbes, inflammatory gut bacteria, poor diet, and stress (including physical trauma such as accidents, ultraviolet radiation, and EMFs; and psychological trauma, both the microtrauma of living in our modern world and big traumas such as severe illness, abuse, or neglect). It is not only what we have too much of that causes inflammation but also what we are lacking: protective anti-inflammatory, whole, phytonutrient-rich foods; optimal levels of vitamins and minerals; exercise; optimal sleep; deep restorative practices like meditation, yoga, prayer, and breath work; connection; love; community; and meaning and purpose.

Inflammation accelerates in what is called a *feed-forward cycle*. It is like a wildfire that spreads throughout the body, wreaking havoc on every cell and organ. Zombie cells are a big part of why inflammation increases as we age. The key is cooling the fire. Doctors today must become inflammologists, detectives rooting out the source of the fire that negatively impacts all seven of the core biological systems. How do we create a virtuous cycle of healing, repair, rejuvenation, and renewal?

The key to healthy aging is a life that enhances the immune system's ability to fight infection and cancer while not overheating and creating low-level chronic inflammation. To cool off inflammation and strengthen your immune system, you need to avoid toxins, allergens, microbial imbalances (dysbiosis), chronic stress, and a sedentary lifestyle. And you need to eat an anti-inflammatory diet, get the optimal levels of nutrients, and have the right balance of movement, sleep, stress reduction, community, and connection.

The Young Forever Program is designed to eliminate or limit the things that cause inflammation while activating your anti-inflammatory pathways.

CORE SYSTEM 3: ENERGY—OUR CELLULAR POWER PLANTS

Without energy, every cellular function becomes problematic, as you learned about in hallmark 7. Learning how to clean up, repair, protect, increase the number of, and optimize the function of mitochondria is the key to healthy aging.

Each one of your 30-plus trillion cells has hundreds to thousands of mitochondria, with concentrations highest in tissues that require the most energy, like your brain and heart. These mitochondria convert the food you eat and oxygen you breathe into energy called *adenosine triphosphate,* or *ATP,* which your body uses to drive nearly every biochemical process. One by-product of this reaction is the creation of a small amount of free radicals, or reactive oxygen species (ROS).

Some ROS is normal and needed for cell homeostasis, but as we age, mitochondrial quality and quantity naturally decline. Mitochondria end up producing too little ATP and too much ROS, which contributes to damage and inflammation that can snowball throughout the body. Ideally, your mitochondria would function optimally to create energy until they are replaced by new, young mitochondria.

Instead, we see that with biological aging and certain diseases, mito-chondria can slowly decline in function, mucking up your cells. If your mitochondria are not functioning well, it's like having a sluggish engine. Cleaning and tuning up your mitochondria are key to healthy aging and longevity.

Many of the advances in longevity science, such as calorie restriction; time-restricted eating; fasting; exercise; NAD+ therapy, rapamy-cin, metformin, and various phytochemicals such as resveratrol, fisetin, and quercetin; cold therapy; red-light therapy; hyperbaric oxygen; ozone; and hypoxia or low oxygen states (which we will cover in Chapter 10), work through improving the number and function of your mitochondria, no matter how old they are.

The Young Forever Program is designed to repair and supercharge your mitochondria.

CORE SYSTEM 4: BIOTRANSFORMATION AND ELIMINATION—DETOXIFICATION

The word "detox" makes many people think of rehab or a fad diet. But your biological detoxification system is quite sophisticated, pro-cessing and removing internal waste and environmental toxins. Imag-ine if your sewer line backed up but you kept using the toilet anyway. Not too pretty. Something similar can happen in your body. If your liver can't process waste, your body turns yellow (called jaundice) and you would die without a liver transplant. If your kidneys stop doing their job, you would get very sick and would die in a week without dialysis. If your colon gets permanently stopped up, well, you probably don't even want to think about what would happen!

Thankfully, our bodies are equipped with sophisticated detoxifica-tion and cleaning systems—our liver, kidneys, lungs, skin, and diges-tive and lymph systems. The liver is an extraordinary organ that takes up toxins, transforms them, and excretes them through your bile into your gut to be eliminated. The kidneys filter waste from your blood and turn it into urine. The lungs get rid of carbon dioxide, the

metabolic waste made by processing food and oxygen in your mitochondria that must be released from your body. The skin allows you to
sweat out toxins. The digestive system removes waste from food and
drink, passing the remains out your colon. The lymph system cleans
up all the metabolic waste excreted by your cells and toxins produced
in the process of living.

Unfortunately, the toxic burden in the twenty-first century often
overwhelms our body's detoxification systems, resulting in disease.
This leads to illness, shortens our health span, and decreases our life
span. Sadly, most physicians learn nothing about the effects of chronic
exposure to low-level environmental toxins. Strangely, even though
the medical literature confirms the link between toxins and most of
our chronic diseases, most doctors don't address it. For example, Parkinson's disease has a well-recognized link to environmental toxins.
Farmers have the highest rates from exposure to pesticides. Arsenic,
pesticides, and bisphenol-A cause diabetes.[3] And in one study, people
with a lead level over 2 mcg/dL ("normal" is considered under 10, but
science is clear that even very low levels of metals can be toxic) had
dramatically higher risks for heart attack, stroke, and death — higher
even than the risks attributed to elevated cholesterol. And about 40
percent of the population has lead levels above this number.[4] Yet when
was the last time your doctor checked your lead levels along with your
cholesterol? Lead overload is something easy to treat with the right
foods, nutrients, and sometimes medication if necessary.

I had mercury poisoning in my thirties. It left me debilitated with
chronic fatigue syndrome. Every one of my body's systems broke
down. My gut was a mess, with bloating and diarrhea for years. My
immune system reacted to everything, including food and environmental allergens, leaving me with rashes and sores in my mouth. My
mitochondria were damaged, causing my muscles to literally break
down. My hormones, including thyroid and adrenal hormones, were
out of whack. My brain felt like it was broken, with severe brain
fog and insomnia. It wasn't until I activated and supported all my
detoxification systems and was treated with chelation therapy (using

medication to bind metals) to remove the overload of toxins that I was able to recover.

The good news is that functional medicine is great at identifying your body's burden of toxins and upregulating your detoxification systems. I call it activating the 4-P system: process (liver), poop, pee, perspire. In the Young Forever Program you will learn how to test for and identify your toxic burden, reduce your exposures, and super-charge your detoxification system.

CORE SYSTEM 5: COMMUNICATION—HORMONES, NEUROTRANSMITTERS, AND CELL-SIGNALING MOLECULES

The body has a finely orchestrated system of communication and feedback loops that keeps our biology functioning optimally. We have a myriad of human messenger molecules (in addition to the thousands of molecules in food) that provide instructions governing nearly every function of our body. These messengers include hormones, neu-rotransmitters, peptides (messenger proteins that control many of our biological functions), and many other cell-signaling molecules. When these communication systems are in balance, we are healthy and happy; when they're not, we are off-kilter, and our health degrades. As we age, these systems malfunction because of all the harmful inputs we have discussed or the lack of ingredients we need to thrive. Much of the dysfunction is secondary to other insults, such as poor diet, nutrient deficiencies, stress, environmental toxins, dysbiosis in the gut, allergens, and infections. Addressing those factors and adding in the ingredients for health help to reset our hormone, neurotransmit-ter, and cell messenger systems.

As we age, predictable, mostly avoidable (and reversible) changes occur—insulin resistance or pre-diabetes, low thyroid function, ele-vated stress hormones such as cortisol, lower adrenal hormones such as DHEA, lower growth hormone and testosterone in men and estrogen and progesterone in women, and changes in our neurotransmitters. All hormonal systems worsen as we age, but not inevitably.

Menopause and andropause are both real phenomena, but their impacts are magnified by our lifestyle and environment. When our hormones are out of balance, they cause tremendous suffering and accelerate aging. The good news is that the Young Forever Program, with hormonal optimization therapy when appropriate, can slow or stop many of the changes we see with age.

Your hormones are like a symphony. Each hormone acts like a different instrument in the orchestra, interpreting a signal from the conductor and then responding appropriately. All your hormones work together. When they are out of tune you feel bad, get sick, and age faster.

The four horsemen of the apocalypse of aging are high insulin, low thyroid function, high cortisol, and low sex hormones (testosterone, estrogen, progesterone). The key to balanced hormones is to reduce the biological insults and take advantage of the interventions now available to support optimal hormone function, including diet, exercise, stress reduction, phytochemicals and herbs, and, when needed, bioidentical hormone therapy for men and women. Some may also need bioidentical thyroid replacement and adrenal support with DHEA. Changes in hormones are such a key part of aging. Let's dig in a little deeper.

Insulin

Insulin resistance from biological aging now affects nine in ten Americans, who fall somewhere along the spectrum of pre-diabetes to full-blown type 2 diabetes (see "The Insulin-Signaling Pathway" under "Hallmark 1" in Chapter 4).[6] Insulin resistance is the single biggest hormonal disorder we face. The main cause: our high-sugar, high-starch diet and sedentary lifestyle. Too much insulin creates a domino effect. It drives all those excess calories into belly-fat cells. These are not regular fat cells; they are dangerous, angry cells that produce messenger molecules that increase hunger, slow metabolism, prevent fat burning, spike inflammation, lower testosterone, increase estrogen in men and both estrogen and testosterone in women, and increase stress hormones (e.g., cortisol). They also adversely impact all the longevity switches (insulin signaling, mTOR, sirtuins, and AMPK), accelerating aging. We don't just get fat bellies, producing a flood of harmful hormones, neurotransmitters, and cytokines that age us rapidly; our modern Western diet and lack of exercise cause muscles to become laden with fat. The result: high blood sugar and blood pressure; sexual dysfunction in men; hair loss in women; increased cortisol, which worsens blood sugar and blood pressure and causes further muscle wasting; low growth hormone, impairing sleep, healing, and repair; and systemic inflammation, fueling the wildfire of aging.

Cortisol: The Stress Hormone

Our bodies have a beautifully designed system to handle acute stress. When a danger or stressor occurs (real or imagined), our bodies produce a flood of compounds that get us ready to fight or flee. Our adrenal glands pump out cortisol and adrenaline. Our heart pumps faster, our blood clots more easily, our mind gets sharp, and glucose floods our bloodstream to fuel our escape from danger. It's a great system designed for acute stress. However, modern life is rife with chronic stressors. Processed food and sugar and starch, toxins, our stressful culture, social media, economic disparities, childhood traumas, and social isolation all register in the body in the same way as acute stress. Long-term elevations in cortisol are a disaster for health and longevity. The consequences: obesity, diabetes, cancer, heart disease, dementia, autoimmunity, depression, sarcopenia...the list goes on. Incorporating daily practices of stress reduction is an essential part of creating health and living a long, vibrant life.

Thyroid Hormones

Your thyroid is an essential part of your metabolic health. Low thyroid function slows everything down. The result: fatigue; weight gain; depression; memory loss; low sex drive; dry skin, hair, and nails; constipation; elevated cholesterol; muscle cramps; and an increased risk of heart attacks. An overactive thyroid speeds everything up. The result:

rapid heart rate, high blood pressure, weight loss, insomnia, anxiety. Low thyroid function affects one in five women and one in ten men. Environmental toxins, gluten, stress, and nutrient deficiencies all contribute to sluggish thyroid function. Thyroid hormones are produced in the thyroid gland and depend on the right nutrients to function properly, including amino acids (tyrosine), selenium, vitamin D, and iodine. Tuning up your thyroid is key to a long and healthy life.

Sex Hormones: Estrogen, Progesterone, Testosterone

Shifts in sex hormones are normal with aging. But these changes are often more extreme today because of our modern diet, lifestyle, and exposure to hormone-disrupting toxins. Keeping your sex hormones optimized as you age is essential to feeling and being strong, active, and even sexually active throughout your whole life.

Estrogen is found in the highest quantities in women, but men also make estrogen. Formed primarily in the ovaries or testes, estrogen is important for women's menstrual cycles and for bone formation and health, blood clotting, skin and hair, mood, sex drive, and reproductive function. Estrogen levels increase with puberty and decrease with age.

Progesterone is produced by the ovaries and adrenals in women and the testes and adrenals in men. While progesterone is found in much higher quantities in women, it is important for men as well. Progesterone supports reproduction, ovulation, pregnancy, and sperm count and quality. It also allows the body to calm down, relax, and sleep. Progesterone is required to form testosterone.

Testosterone is also produced by both men and women, though men have much higher levels. It's important for sperm production, motivation, sex drive and libido, muscle mass, bone health, exercise recovery, and strengthening the adrenal glands (important for cortisol regulation). It's also neuroprotective. Low testosterone levels have been associated with obstructive sleep apnea for both men and women. Testosterone production decreases with age and menopause but should not be so low that it accelerates muscle loss and limits sexual function (for both men and women).

The key to balancing hormones is to reduce the biological insults that disrupt hormone balance and incorporate behaviors and treatments that optimize hormone function, including diet, exercise, stress reduction, phytochemicals and herbs, and, when needed, bioidentical hormone therapy for men and women. Fine-tuning and optimizing all these hormonal systems is an essential part of a healthy aging strategy and the Young Forever Program.

CORE SYSTEM 6: TRANSPORT—OPTIMIZING CIRCULATION AND LYMPHATIC FLOW

Taking Care of Our Blood Vessels

How do all the messages get to where they need to go for the body's optimal functioning? How does the food you eat, and all the magic it contains, find the right receptors to act upon? How does the body clear waste? Through our transportation systems: our circulatory system (the blood vessels and heart) and our lymphatic system, a parallel set of vessels that clears metabolic waste from your tissues and sends it to the liver and kidneys for removal.

Our body contains about 100,000 miles (160,000km) of blood vessels, enough to go around the Earth about two and a half times. But these vessels are not just inert tubes that carry blood; they are also immune and hormonal organs and require the right diet to function optimally. The lining of the vessels is called the *endothelium*. When it is dysfunctional it gets stiff and can cause high blood pressure, and it can lay down dysfunctional cholesterol and cause hardening of the arteries. The result? Cardiovascular disease, the number one killer worldwide.

Many of the key hallmarks of aging, including inflammaging, damaged proteins, and altered nutrient sensing (insulin resistance), cause damage to your blood vessels and are at the root of heart disease. If your blood vessels are sick, so are your heart, brain, and every other organ and system in your body. Heart disease is largely caused by insulin resistance. The consequences: heart attacks, high blood pressure, strokes, amputations in diabetics, and even dementia. Our approach has been to bypass the problem, literally, with heart bypass operations and angioplasty or stents, or to lower cholesterol with medication. But none of these addresses the root causes of the problem. Cholesterol is not the problem. Heart disease is triggered when inflammation and hormonal changes turn cholesterol into fragile plaques that coat our arteries.

Ninety percent of heart disease can be prevented with a healthy diet, exercise, and not smoking.[5] Heart disease, it turns out, is an inflammatory and hormonal disease. What causes the most inflammation and hormonal chaos (direct downstream effects of insulin resistance)? Our diet. While environmental toxins, stress, our microbiome, and genetics all play a role, our diet is the biggest driver of cardiovascular disease. It is the high-sugar, high-starch, low-fiber, nutrient-depleted, phytonutrient-poor, ultraprocessed-food, damaged-fat diet. Eating a whole foods anti-inflammatory, low-glycemic, high-fiber, phytonutrient- and omega-3-rich diet is key to protecting yourself from the ravages of heart disease.

Bottom line: Optimizing diet and lifestyle (exercise, stress management, sleep) for longevity, a process laid out in the Young Forever Program, will address most of the risks for heart disease.

Lymphatic Flow: Our Other Transport System

A much-neglected aspect of our health is our lymphatic system. We can't see it, we can't touch it, it doesn't show up on an X-ray, but it is working all the time to clear metabolic waste, the by-products of all our cellular processes, from our tissues. Our lymphatic system absorbs fats from the gut and transports them into our general circulation, and brings white blood cells to and from lymph nodes to help us fight infection and cancer. It also connects our immune system to our circulation because the lymph vessels empty into the veins that go into your heart. A high intake of processed foods, low levels of nutrients, and a lack of physical activity can throw it out of balance and contribute to arthritis, headaches, digestive and skin disorders, excess weight, and fatigue. When our lymphatic system is not functioning well, we retain fluid and are puffy, swollen, and sluggish.

The heart pumps blood around our blood vessels, but your lymphatic vessels need movement—muscle activity and breathing—to pump the waste fluid for detoxification through your liver and kidneys. There are lots of ways to improve lymphatic circulation, including exercise, lymphatic massage, hot and cold showers, steam and saunas followed by cold dips, dry brushing, lots of hydration, and deep breathing. Of course, what you eat matters too. The Young Forever Program is designed to optimize both your circulatory and lymphatic systems.

CORE SYSTEM 7: STRUCTURAL HEALTH AND IMBALANCES—FROM MUSCLE AND BONES TO CELLS AND TISSUES

How do you build a house of health and longevity? Not with straw but with brick. Our musculoskeletal system—our meat suit—determines our quality of life. If it is weak and arthritic and frail, we can't do what we love, whether it is dance during sunrise or play with our grandchildren. If we eat junk, we get junk bones, muscles, and tissues. If we don't move our bodies as they were designed—run and lift and stretch—they gradually weaken and start to disintegrate. Do you want to be made from high-fructose corn syrup, white flour, and rancid oils, as most Americans are today, or do you want to be constructed from the best raw materials—the highest-quality proteins, fats, vitamins, and minerals?

Your structure matters—not just to keep you standing straight up and not collapsed in a pile of muscle and bone on the floor. Every part of you has a structure but also a function. If you are made from poor-quality parts, you will create a poorly functioning body. Muscle loss (sarcopenia) and bone loss (osteopenia/osteoporosis) are huge factors in aging and age-related diseases. Muscle is where our metabolism is—low muscle mass means slow metabolism and an increase in diabetes, heart disease, cancer, dementia, inflammation, and aging.

We need the best-quality protein to build muscle and run our body's essential systems. But not all protein is the same. The best type to build muscle is other muscle: animal protein. You can get protein from plant foods, but the quality is lower, and it has lower levels of key amino acids needed to synthesize new muscle, especially the branched-chain amino acids (BCAA) such as leucine, isoleucine, valine, lysine, and sulfur-based amino acids.[7] There are also compounds such as phytates, in plant proteins like beans and nuts, that may impair protein absorption. Rather than being turned into muscle, your body often burns plant proteins as calories. If you are vegan, especially as you age, you need to ensure you get enough protein by increasing the overall volume of protein-rich plant foods, adding protein powders, and supplementing with BCAAs.[8] If you want to eat less meat and include more plant proteins, combining them helps the body use the plant protein rather than burning it. Think chili con carne!

The science is clear: Combining strength training with the right quality protein can both preserve and build muscle mass at any age. In fact, as we age this is not just a good idea; it is imperative if we want to stay agile, strong, functional, and active well over 100 years old.

And don't forget all the vitamins and minerals needed to build tissues, muscles, and bones, including vitamin D, vitamin K, calcium, magnesium, and more. For some, like me, who have suffered from injuries, regenerative medicine (which we explore in Chapter 11) that uses stem cells, exosomes, placental matrix (which is filled with healing compounds), ozone, and peptides can be very helpful in renewing and rebuilding damaged joints and tissues.

But it is not only your muscles and bones that determine how you age. It is the health of your cells. What are your cells made of? What you eat. Every cell membrane is the docking station for all the thousands of chemical messengers communicating with your cells. Every membrane is made of fat. If it is made of Trex, it is stiff, hard, and dysfunctional. If it is made of omega-3 fats, say, from sardines, it is soft, pliable, and able to receive all those cellular messengers.

Imagine building your house out of rotten wood and disintegrating bricks. You wouldn't do it. Why would you build your body from defective ingredients? You need the best-quality fats—your brain is 60 percent fat, your nerve coverings are all made from fat, every one of your 30 trillion cells is wrapped in a little fatty membrane. Do you really want to make these from oxidized, damaged, refined oils in your French fries? Next time you chomp down on something, ask yourself if you are fine with those nasty ingredients becoming part of you for the long term. If not, don't eat it. Find the best-quality ingredients you can, ingredients that help you thrive.

The Young Forever Program is designed to help you build a strong foundation for healthy muscles, bones, and cells.

You have just journeyed through the world of the human body—how it works, what's needed for its proper function, and how to create health and a long, vibrant life. In this exploration of our body's underlying biological systems, you had a quick glimpse into the complexity of how everything is connected. My hope was to give you a taste of the magic of our bodies and their intimate dance with what we eat, what we do, and how we live. Understanding how to optimize these systems is key to addressing the hallmarks of aging, reversing disease, and aging backward. It is the foundation of the Young Forever Program, laid out in Part III.

Chapter 7

Eating for Longevity

Let food be thy medicine and medicine be thy food.
— ATTRIBUTED TO HIPPOCRATES

The food you eat can be either the safest and most powerful form of medicine or the slowest form of poison.
— ANN WIGMORE

The foundational principles of staying healthy have not changed in thousands of years. Sadly, they are mostly ignored. But the good news is we have the power to return to those principles that will reverse disease and extend our health span and life span, no matter when we start. The ancient principles of longevity practiced in places like Sardinia and Ikaria help us build the framework for a long, healthy life. The new science of longevity has given us a deeper understanding of aging and how to literally become biologically younger as we grow chronologically older. Following these principles will not only prevent disease and extend life but make you feel younger and more vibrant and alive right away.

Optimizing our exposome rests on addressing the fundamental lifestyle factors that are the foundation of functional medicine—factors that help balance every one of the body's core biological networks and address many of the hallmarks of aging. What are they?

Optimal nutrition, exercise and movement, sleep and relaxation, stress management, and relationships and community. The Young Forever Program starts with these powerful tools. These can be enough to achieve your goals. Sometimes more work is needed to address deeper layers of dysfunction, such as a severe gut imbalance or high load of toxins or hormonal imbalances or infections or traumas. Let's get started with one of the most powerful tools we have at our disposal right now: what and how we eat.

NUTRITIONAL OPTIMIZATION

What is the optimal longevity diet? Should you be a vegetarian like the Seventh-Day Adventists from the Loma Linda Blue Zone, or should you be a carnivore eating primarily bison, which allowed the Plains Indians to have the highest number of centenarians at the turn of the 1900s? Is it beans and grains or meat and dairy? Should we eat vegan or paleo? Raw foods or lectin-free? Fruitarian or breatharian? Low-carb or high-carb? Low-fat or high-fat?

If you are wondering what to eat for lunch, you are not alone. The confusion wrought by difficult-to-interpret nutritional science, compounded by the ideological diet wars, is enough to make you give up and eat that doughnut. I have written a few books to help clarify the science — what we know and what we don't — and help you choose a way of eating that is personalized to your body and culture and beliefs. For a deeper dive into what to eat, read *The Pegan Diet* and *Food: What the Heck Should I Eat?*

The foundational principles of eating for health and longevity are not in dispute and can be summarized in Michael Pollan's pithy aphorism, "Eat food. Not too much. Mostly plants." Let's unpack that: Eat real food. Not ultraprocessed, food-like substances, but foods unaltered by modern agriculture. Don't overeat, which is easier to do if you eat nutrient-dense food that gives your body all the protein, fat, fiber, vitamins, minerals, and phytonutrients it needs. And eat mostly plants because they contain thousands of medicinal, life-extending phytonutrients. After that it can get a bit more complicated and nuanced. What do we eat, when do we eat, how often should we eat? Do our needs change as we age?

In Chapter 4, in the discussion of nutrient-sensing pathways, one of the hallmarks of aging, you learned how to eat to turn on your longevity switches. These principles are embedded in the Young Forever Longevity Diet.

NUTRITIONAL PERSONALIZATION: BALANCING YOUR SEVEN CORE SYSTEMS

The number one intervention to prevent, treat, and reverse disease, and more importantly to create health, is food. Think of food as your *farm*acy. Literally. Food is not *like* medicine. It *is* medicine. It works on your biology in wondrous and complex ways that are often far more powerful than pharmaceuticals. Just as there is not one drug to treat every disease or symptom, there is not one food that works for everything. Food is information that regulates every function of your body, all the core biological systems we described in Chapter 6. It does so in real time, with rapid results. It's essential to support each of those systems by knowing what foods help and harm. Following are the dietary strategies to rebuild and balance your seven core systems.

Optimizing Core System 1: Gut Health and the Microbiome

Turns out the microbiome, the magical kingdom of microbes living within you, may be the most important organ in your body, orchestrating every function of your biology. Just as the right foods keep your inner garden healthy, the wrong foods create havoc, often feeding the bugs you don't want—the bugs that drive inflammation and leaky gut.

Bad bugs grow for two reasons: not enough of the foods that feed the good guys and too many foods that feed the bad ones. Gluten is the biggest offender. Today's modern hybridized dwarf wheat contains far more inflammatory proteins than ancient wheat and results in a leaky gut. Even in those not gluten-sensitive, eating a lot of gluten tends to disrupt gut function, not to mention that much of our modern wheat is sprayed at harvest with the weed killer glyphosate.[1] Aside from being a known carcinogen, glyphosate destroys your microbiome. A large national study by the Centers for Disease Control and Prevention found glyphosate in the urine of more than 80 percent of Americans.[2]

Next on the gut-busting list are starch and sugar. The bad guys love it just like you do. It promotes overgrowth of toxic bacteria and yeast. Not fun. And it often leads to that food baby—bloating and feeling miserable—after eating. It also turns out different fats have different impacts on the gut.

The wrong fats cause trouble too. Refined oils (about 10 percent of our calories) trigger something called *metabolic endotoxemia*. In other words, our metabolism is poisoned because of toxic by-products of bad bacteria, leading to obesity and type 2 diabetes.[3] Omega-3 fats do the opposite. It's all about the information in the food.

Next come additives. Some of the worst are the thickeners and emulsifiers in most processed food, including carrageenan and gums. They cause leaky gut and autoimmune diseases.[4]

I would be remiss if I did not mention the gut-busting medications. The worst are the medications used for heartburn and acid reflux, which is mostly caused by diet and occasionally a bacterium called *H. pylori*. Acid-blocking medications such as Prilosec, Prevacid, and Nexium shut off acid production in your stomach, which not only prevents the absorption of B_{12}, zinc, magnesium, and other nutrients, but also leads to overgrowth of bugs in your small intestine and irritable bowel syndrome. Fix one problem but create another! Other drugs, including antibiotics, steroids, hormones, birth control, and anti-inflammatories like Advil, Aleve, and aspirin, result in bad bugs, yeast, and leaky gut.

How do you feed the good bugs? They munch down on the fibers in our food. These are called prebiotics. Fiber-rich foods help keep the garden healthy: vegetables, fruits, nuts, seeds, whole grains, and beans. Certain foods have high levels of prebiotic fibers, including avocados, artichokes, asparagus, berries, peas, chia seeds, and pistachios. Probiotic-rich foods, including traditional fermented foods like sauerkraut, pickles, tempeh, miso, natto, and kimchi, also help support a healthy gut. Some of the exciting discoveries around the microbiome involve the role of polyphenols, the colorful phytonutrients found in plants. The good critters love them and feed on them, and in turn, those bugs protect us. For example, one such bug, *Akkermansia muciniphila,* loves cranberry, pomegranate, and green tea. When it is in abundance, it creates a protective mucous layer in the gut, preventing a leaky gut, autoimmune disease, and even heart disease and diabetes. Turns out this bug is also necessary for certain cancer treatments, such as immunotherapy, to work.[5] Part of the cure for cancer might be feeding *Akkermansia.*

Your gut needs other nutrients, too, to function well and heal: zinc, omega-3 fats, vitamin A, and glutamine. Foods with collagen such as bone broth, and kudzu, a Japanese root, also help your microbiome.

Optimizing Core System 2: Immunity, Defense, and Repair

Our immune system attempts to keep a perfect balance. A little bit of immune activation is good, a lot not so much. While there are other causes of inflammation—toxins, allergens, infections, and stress—for most of us, food plays the greatest role.

A short review. Sugar and starch spike blood sugar, which in turn spikes insulin. Insulin drives sugar and starch to be stored in fat cells called *adipocytes* in your belly and around your organs. This superfat causes metabolic and hormonal chaos and tons of inflammation. As we ingest more and more sugar and starch, we need more and more insulin to overcome the resistance to their effects, just as an alcoholic needs more and more alcohol to get drunk. More insulin, more fat storage, more inflammation. And while sugar drives inflammation, it also suppresses your immune response to infections and fuels bad bugs in your microbiome, resulting in leaky gut and more inflammation.

Fats may be another trigger of inflammation. While the point is still debated in the science, the sheer volume of processed food has increased our intake of refined oils that contain lots of omega-6 fats. We do need them, but you can have too much of a good thing. As hunter-gatherers we consumed our omega-6 fats from nuts and seeds and other plants, not from gallons of industrially produced, solvent-extracted, heat-treated oxidized oils. And we have eliminated most foods containing omega-3 fats, except for seafood. Balance is key; too many omega-6 fats can inhibit the anti-inflammatory effects of omega-3 fats, resulting in inflammation.[6] Best get your omega-6 fats from whole foods such as nuts and seeds or unrefined plant oils. And make sure you get enough omega-3 fats from small wild fish. Population studies show that people who get their omega-6 fats from whole foods do better overall, like the Sardinians and Ikarians, who eat beans, nuts, and seeds, but only extra virgin olive oil and no other refined oils.

Food sensitivities and reactions are another main trigger of inflammation. They create more subtle and generalized inflammation than true allergies, like peanut allergies do, and symptoms are harder to diagnose. The most common foods that trigger reactions are gluten, dairy, grains, beans, soy, eggs, nuts and seeds, and nightshades (tomatoes, peppers, potatoes, aubergines). Healing the gut can reduce or eliminate reactions. This is why an elimination diet is such a powerful tool for anyone with an inflammatory condition. It is why I wrote *The Blood Sugar Solution 10-Day Detox Diet,* a program I have done with thousands of patients to help them heal from myriad diseases. If you are inflamed (see Chapter 13 to help you find out if you have lots of inflammation), following this program for ten days to three months, depending on your level of inflammation, can have profound health benefits. In trials of this diet in more than a thousand people, the average reduction in all symptoms from all diseases was almost 70 percent in just ten days.

The good news is that the polyphenols in plant foods are among nature's best inflammation-fighting compounds. The best place to find these compounds is at the end of the rainbow, the bright pigments and colors found in red, green, yellow, orange, and purple plant foods. Extra virgin olive oil, a nice green color, contains oleocanthal, which has anti-inflammatory properties similar to ibuprofen without all its side effects.

Spices like turmeric, ginger, and rosemary are anti-inflammatory powerhouses. Meat cooked with spices neutralizes any potential inflammation.[7] Mushrooms regulate the immune system and contain anti-cancer compounds. And foods rich in vitamin C, zinc, selenium, and vitamin D strengthen your immunity and slow down inflammation. So a dinner that includes prawns and flaxseeds (zinc), lime juice and coriander (vitamin C), eggs (selenium and vitamin D), and porcini mushrooms (vitamin D) would be a super-immunity meal. Maybe not all those ingredients together, but you get the idea!

Optimizing Core System 3: Energy and Mitochondria

Your mitochondria are like a hybrid engine and can run on two fuel sources: fat and carbohydrates. Most of us fuel our metabolic engines with carbs, a dirty-burning, inefficient fuel, rather than clean-burning fats. Bad fats, including trans fats and oxidized oils (especially from deep-frying), harm our mitochondria. Certain fats called ketones and MCT oil are the preferred fuel to help mitochondria repair, renew, and rebuild. MCT (medium-chain triglyceride) oil is an excellent fuel source for the mitochondria. Unrefined coconut oil contains MCT, or you can buy MCT separately. It burns cleanly and enhances performance if taken before exercise.

Our mitochondria not only need the right fuel; they need the right fuel at the right time. The problem is we just keeping eating all day and most of the night and never give our biology a rest so cells can clean up waste and debris, recycle old parts to make new cells, activate our anti-oxidant and anti-inflammatory systems, get rid of toxic belly fat, increase muscle and bone, and heighten brain function (so we can find the next meal!). When you combine the best foods with the best timing (see

Chapter 14), you activate all the healing mechanisms and supercharge your mitochondria and your life. This is the key to healthy aging.

To produce energy, your mitochondria also need specific nutrients: B vitamins, coenzyme Q10, carnitine, zinc, magnesium, selenium, omega-3 fats, lipoic acid, n-acetylcysteine, vitamin E, vitamin K, sulfur, and others. Foods such as blueberries, pomegranate seeds, grass-fed beef and butter, broccoli, sardines, extra virgin olive oil, avocados, and almonds are great sources of fat and phytonutrients that supercharge your mitochondria.

Learning to feed your mitochondria well, using clean-burning fuels, avoiding sugar and starch, increasing good fats, and ensuring optimal levels of key nutrients[8] can provide a metabolic tune-up.[9] Combining that with minibreaks using time-restricted eating or intermittent fasting (see Chapter 14) can have powerful rejuvenating effects on your health, energy, and longevity.

Optimizing Core System 4: Detoxification

The process of detoxification can be hindered by an overload of processed food, sugar, starch (yes, these culprits are involved in messing up every system in your body), and environmental toxins. Detoxification also requires a host of foods, phytochemicals, protein, vitamins and minerals, fiber, and water to function optimally.

Sadly, we are all toxic waste dumps. Eighty-four thousand chemicals have been introduced into the environment since the industrial revolution. Fewer than 1 percent have been tested for safety. These chemicals cause inflammation and oxidative stress, damage the mitochondria, disrupt our gut function, create hormonal imbalances, and overload our detoxification systems. We ingest five pounds (2.2 kg) of food additives every year,[10] pesticides and weed killers from our food, mercury from our fish, and arsenic and toxins from our water. Sprinkle in a little alcohol and paracetamol (which depletes glutathione, our body's main detoxifying compound) and other meds and our bodies can't keep up — we end up in toxic overload.

The good news is that food contains nearly all the ingredients our bodies need to eliminate waste. Plenty of water helps the kidneys and gut remove waste effectively. Fiber moves waste products through the colon quickly. The liver needs help from phytonutrients in our diet. The food group that best boosts liver detox pathways is the cruciferous vegetable family (broccoli, greens, kale, cabbage, Brussels sprouts), which contains sulfur compounds that enhance the production of glutathione, the most powerful antioxidant in your body. Garlic and onions also provide the sulfur needed for detoxification. The liver also needs adequate levels of B_1, B_2, B_3, B_6, B_{12}, folate, manganese, magnesium, zinc, and selenium found in animal protein, seafood, nuts, seeds, and green vegetables to facilitate all the chemical reactions needed for detoxification. The rich array of phytochemicals found in herbs and spices help the liver detox, too. Curcumin, found in turmeric, helps in detoxification and decreases inflammation.[11]

Adequate amino acids from protein are essential for healthy detox. Green tea is a super detoxifier, which may explain why the Japanese seem to be able to detoxify high mercury levels from sushi. Green tea chelates (binds to) heavy metals. Rosemary, ginger, coriander, dandelion greens, parsley, lemon peel, watercress, burdock root, and artichokes are all powerful detoxifying foods that should be consumed on a regular basis.

High-quality protein, phytonutrients, and vitamin- and mineral-rich foods, along with lots of fiber and fresh clean water, keep our detox system humming and our toxic load low.

Optimizing Core System 5: Communication and Hormones

If there is one single cause of accelerated aging and diseases of aging, it is this: sugar and starch (especially flour) and the resulting metabolic chaos and insulin resistance. You might be tired of hearing this over and over, but eliminating sugar and flour is the single biggest thing you can do to improve your health and extend your life, not only for your hormones and neurotransmitters, but also for every other core system.

Women need to pay special attention to balancing their hormones because we live in a hormone-disrupting world that causes or worsens menopause, PMS, and female cancers and drives excess estrogen in the body. Too much sugar, low-fiber diets, nutritional deficiencies, alcohol, xenoestrogens (pesticides, plastics, and environmental chemicals that mimic estrogen), stress, and lack of exercise all drive hormonal imbalances. Women benefit from including in their diet non–GMO traditional soy foods such as miso, natto, tempeh, and tofu; flaxseeds; cruciferous vegetables; and lots of fiber.

What we eat also impacts our thyroid function. Low thyroid function can be triggered by gluten, too many raw kale smoothies (raw cruciferous veggies can block thyroid function), and diets low in zinc, selenium, vitamin D, and iodine. Adding foods rich in zinc (meat, seeds, nuts), selenium (sardines and Brazil nuts), vitamin D (egg yolks, porcini mushrooms, and herring), and iodine (seaweed and fish) can help optimize thyroid function.

Our brain and neurotransmitters are also highly impacted by our diet. Whole new fields of psychiatry have emerged that recognize the power of food to influence brain function. Stanford has a department of metabolic psychiatry. Harvard has a department of nutritional and lifestyle psychiatry. Many studies demonstrate the impact of dietary change on dementia.[19] Ketogenic diets have been shown to improve cognition and function in Alzheimer's patients.[20] Harvard psychiatrists have used ketogenic diets to put schizophrenia into remission.[21] Studies show that simply swapping out the processed sugary, starchy foods for whole foods is effective in treating depression—in fact, 400 percent better in treating depression than the SAD diet (standard American diet), which the control group remained on.[22] Maybe we should call a whole foods diet the GLAD diet!

Bottom line. To paraphrase President Clinton, "It's the sugar, stupid."

Optimizing Core System 6: Circulation and Lymphatic Health

Your transportation systems—circulatory and lymphatic—clear the metabolic waste from your tissues and return it to the heart to be cleansed by the liver and kidneys. What drives dysfunction in blood vessels and lymphatic flow and promotes heart disease? You guessed it.

Our modern industrial, processed, high-starch, high-sugar, and high-refined-fats inflammatory diet, which is low in protective medicinal foods. A single fast-food meal hurts blood vessels.[12] Much of the adverse effects can be offset by consuming phytonutrients[13] and antioxidants.[14] Eating a nutrient-dense whole foods diet rich in phytonutrients will prevent the damage in the first place.[15]

The other important foods for vascular health are those that increase nitric oxide, which increases blood flow. Your body needs the amino acid arginine to produce nitric oxide, and the best food sources are pumpkin seeds, sesame seeds, walnuts, almonds, turkey breast, soybeans, and seaweed. Omega-3 fats from wild fish also help improve endothelial function (the function of the lining of the blood vessels) and prevent dangerous clotting.[16] The heart-healthy benefits of olive oil come from the effect of polyphenols on endothelial function and reducing blood vessel inflammation.[17]

High blood pressure leads to heart attacks, heart failure, strokes, and kidney failure. But what leads to high blood pressure? While genetics, salt sensitivity, environmental pollution, and heavy metals are factors, for most people, high blood pressure is driven by insulin resistance. If you have belly fat, it is likely causing your high blood pressure. If you are like about 40 percent of Americans, you are also magnesium deficient.[18] And low magnesium leads to high blood pressure. Magnesium relaxes blood vessels. Stress, alcohol, caffeine, and sugar all deplete magnesium. It is found in foods we eat too little of: nuts, seeds, beans, and greens.

The heart pumps blood through your blood vessels, but your lymphatic vessels need movement, muscle activity, and breathing to pump waste fluid back into your heart. There are lots of ways to improve lymphatic circulation, which we will cover in Chapter 17, but what you eat matters, too. Common culprits that tend to impair lymphatic function are processed foods, dairy, sugar, sweeteners, and excess salt. Yet many foods help improve lymphatic function, including green leafy vegetables, ground flaxseeds, chia seeds, avocados, garlic, nuts, seaweed, citrus fruits, and cranberries. Phytochemically rich herbs can also help, like echinacea, astragalus, coriander, and parsley.

Optimizing Core System 7: Muscles, Bones, and Cells — What We Are Made Of

We don't just create new cells, organs, tissues, skin, muscles, bone, and brain cells from thin air. The raw materials come from food. Our structure—how strong it is and how well it functions—depends on what we provide as building blocks: the proteins, fats, and minerals we ingest. You might be surprised to learn that carbs are not essential nutrients. Yet our Western processed diet is 50 to 60 percent carbohydrates, and most of those come from low-quality refined starches and sugars. If those carbs aren't essential for our structure, where do they go? We burn some, but most get turned into dangerous disease-causing belly fat, which triggers the hallmarks of aging.

If you are made of poor-quality parts, you will create a poorly functioning body. Muscle loss and bone loss are huge factors in aging and age-related diseases. Muscle is where metabolism happens—low muscle mass equals slow metabolism and worse. Poor-quality muscles marbled with fat lead to diabetes, inflammation, and aging.

The body makes most of its important molecules from protein. Not all protein is the same. The best type of protein to build muscle is other muscle: animal protein. Yes, protein also exists in many plant foods, but the quality is not the same and it doesn't have as many of the essential amino acids that your body needs to create new muscle, especially the branched-chain amino acids (BCAA), such as leucine, iso-leucine, valine, lysine, and sulfur-based amino acids.[23] There are also compounds such as phytates in plant proteins like beans and nuts that impair protein absorption. (But don't take that to mean you should avoid beans and nuts; you just need the right balance.) If you are vegan, especially as you age, you need to ensure you get branched-chain amino acids by increasing the overall volume of protein-rich plant foods, adding protein powders, and supplementing with BCAA—or if you are not vegan, it might be helpful to boost your protein using protein powders such as goat whey.[24]

And don't forget all the vitamins and minerals needed to build tissues, muscles, and bones, including vitamin D, vitamin K, calcium, magnesium, and boron.

PHYTOCHEMICAL HORMESIS AND LONGEVITY: EAT STRESSED FOODS

The Rockefeller Foundation is spending $200 million to create a periodic table of the tens of thousands of potentially beneficial medicinal molecules, called *phytochemicals,* found in the plant kingdom (see the Periodic Table of Food Initiative; foodperiodictable.org). Locked in these plant molecules are powerful medicines that have the potential to prevent and reverse disease and extend life. You might wonder why plants would care about our health. They don't. These molecules are part of their own defense, protection, and communications systems. Many of them are poisons designed to deter predators and create stress resistance against harsh environments and other dangers, such as ultraviolet radiation. These compounds are highest in wild plants, then regeneratively raised foods, and then organic foods. They are found in very small amounts in industrially grown vegetables, grains, and beans that have been bred for yield, starch content, and resistance to drought, pesticides, and herbicides. The result: flavorless foods with higher sugar content, lower protein, and far fewer vitamins, minerals, and phytochemicals.

These compounds—like alkaloids, polyphenols, and terpenes—can be toxic in high doses, but when consumed in small amounts they produce a little beneficial stress to our system. That stress is called *hormesis,* a phenomenon that also occurs during fasting, saunas, cold plunges, exercise, and more. What doesn't kill us makes us stronger; hormesis is essential to activating our innate healing systems. We will cover hormesis in more detail in Chapter 10. But know now that if we eat stressed plants, our bodies respond by optimizing pathways for health and longevity.

The good news is that true flavor in foods (not flavoring added by the industrial food system) always follows the phytochemical richness of the plant or animal. A tiny wild strawberry bursts with flavor and the age-reversing phytochemical fisetin. The large, starchy, crush-proof industrial strawberry may look good but tastes bland. Organic produce contains 10 to 50 percent more phytochemicals than conventional produce.[25]

Dan Barber, the renowned chef of Blue Hill at Stone Barns, went in search of flavor in vegetables but found much has been bred out in modern crops. He founded Row 7 Seeds to create new versions of vegetables, almost reverse engineering them to their wild or heirloom states to produce more flavorful varietals. The side effect: He enhanced the phytochemical richness of the vegetables.

We humans are biologically lazy. Throughout our evolution we have borrowed these compounds to fill in critical gaps in our biochemistry and physiology. Small doses of these compounds produce little challenges to our system, gently encouraging repair, healing, and longevity and helping us build resilience in the face of life's stresses.

While the lack of phytochemicals in our diet from fruits and vegetables may not cause a true deficiency disease like scurvy or rickets, a long-term lack manifests in chronic disease and a shortened life span. We need these compounds to thrive and to activate healing and longevity pathways. I like to call this relationship between plants and humans *symbiotic phytoadaptation;* others called it *xenohormesis* or *phytohormesis.* The only thing that all nutrition scientists agree on is that health and longevity are directly tied to the number of fruits and vegetables in your diet (and no, French fries and ketchup don't count!).

As we have seen with calorie restriction, fasting, and exercise, phytochemicals induce a set of responses in the body that protect us from aging by activating or inhibiting critical processes, including autophagy, DNA repair, and powerful antioxidant enzymes. They work by creating a small stress, then stimulating the body to activate its systems for stress resistance. Phytochemicals such as alkaloids, polyphenols, and terpenoids, found in plants, and polysaccharides, found in fungi, work through the same pathways we have discussed, including nutrient-sensing mechanisms, mTOR, insulin-signaling pathways, sirtuins, AMPK, and our own built-in antioxidant defense systems. They also seem to work by improving gut health, preventing leaky gut and feeding the good bugs, and increasing production of short-chain fatty acids, critical energy sources for intestinal cells. These short-chain fats are also absorbed and reduce systemic inflammation.[26] For instance, some phytochemicals, like sulforaphane, from broccoli,[27] or epigallo-catechin gallate (EGCG),[28] a polyphenol found in green tea, reduce oxidative stress by activating a pathway called Nrf2, which turns on the production of our own antioxidant enzymes. And experimental evidence shows that the polyamine spermidine, found in human sperm cells but also in mushrooms, aged cheese, and soybeans (notably in natto, a fermented soybean preparation) and available as a dietary supplement, extends life span in mice and people.[29]

We long thought it was the antioxidants found in plants that provided the benefit from eating fruits and vegetables, but it turns out that phytochemicals are the heroes. There is a fine dance of oxidation in the body. We need a little but not too much to regulate many important cellular processes. Overdosing on antioxidants may have a deleterious effect. The phytochemical richness of your diet reduces overall death rates and lowers heart disease, dementia, and cancer. Coffee, one of the highest sources of polyphenols in our modern diet (mostly because we don't eat enough vegetables), is associated with lower death rates,[30] as is the Mediterranean diet, which is naturally high in phytochemical-rich foods.[31] Many plant and fungal compounds, including berberine, curcumin, fisetin, quercetin, resveratrol, and silibinin, from milk thistle, can extend life span and health span in model organisms such as yeasts, nematodes, fruit flies, and rodents.

All in all, these plant compounds pack a powerful health-promoting longevity punch.

The Phytochemical Immuno-Rejuvenating Power of an Ancient Food

A newly rediscovered plant, Himalayan Tartary buckwheat, an ancient gluten-free grain (actually a flower) grown in harsh, cold climates with bad soils and little water in the Himalayas, survives by producing very high amounts of phytochemicals.[32] This buckwheat may be the world's most powerful superfood, with more than 132 phytonutrients, higher protein, less starch, and more vitamins and minerals than any other grain product. It contains high levels of quercetin, luteolin, and something called *hobamine* (2-hydroxy-benzyl amine; aka 2-HOBA), a rare age-reversing phytochemical so far found nowhere else in nature. The phytochemicals may work in unique ways through a process of immune rejuvenation and mitochondrial rejuvenation.[33] Using the phytochemicals in this buckwheat plant as a supplement or in an upgraded version of buckwheat pancakes or soba noodles can help you reset your immune system and improve mitochondrial function.

PHYTOCHEMICALS AND THE GUT MICROBIOME

In 2016, after a dose of an antibiotic for an infected root canal, my gut went haywire. I developed a life-threatening infection called *Clostridium difficile,* which turned into full-blown colitis. My normal gut-repair tricks didn't work. It was then that I discovered the true power of polyphenols on the microbiome. Turns out we aren't the only ones who benefit from phytochemicals in our diet. The trillions of critters in our gut also thrive when we feed them the right phytochemicals. I developed a severe leaky gut and had low levels of an important keystone species called *Akkermansia muciniphila* that is responsible for the mucous layer lining our gut, which we need to protect us from leaky gut. It loves cranberry, pomegranate, olives, prickly pear, and green tea! Stimulating the growth of just this one bacterium is associated with reduction in body weight, oxidative stress, and intestinal and liver inflammation and improved insulin sensitivity.[34] It is so important that those with low levels may not respond to immunotherapy, one of the greatest advances in cancer care.

Other compounds also keep your gut healthy. Resveratrol prevents leaky gut and reverses dysbiosis. Quercetin and ginseng do the same thing. A beautiful symbiosis exists when we feed our microbiome phytochemicals. They thrive, and the good bacteria produce healing compounds that enhance our own health, such as *urolithin A*.

A Post-Biotic Muscle-Building, Energy-Enhancing Polyphenol: Urolithin A

Another promising "longevity molecule," urolithin A, is produced when certain gut bacteria (often depleted in modern humans) are exposed to the phytochemicals in pomegranate, berries, and walnuts. Sadly, our modern microbiome can't produce this metabolite of pomegranate. Since it is produced by gut bacteria, then absorbed by the body, it is called a post-biotic. This molecule addresses two key hallmarks of aging: declining mitochondrial function and number and inflammation. Urolithin A induces mitophagy, or the cleaning up of old mitochondria, as well as the production of more mitochondria. It also seems to lower systemic inflammation as measured by lower C-reactive protein levels.

A recent randomized controlled trial in middle-aged overweight adults found that it worked like exercise in a pill. After four months of taking a supplement form of urolithin A, the participants increased leg muscle strength by 12 percent, improved VO_2 max (a measure of aerobic fitness) by 10 percent, and improved physical performance measures such as distance walked and the strength of the muscles—all while doing not a lick of exercise.[35] Since sarcopenia is such a critical feature of aging, a supplement that can reverse it and improve muscle function as we age is a significant finding. Using sophisticated techniques looking at gene expression, changes in protein signatures of longevity, and metabolomics (the metabolites made by your body or by gut bacteria) with blood tests and muscle biopsies, the researchers were able to map the health-promoting longevity effects of these ancient polyphenol post-biotic molecules in exquisite detail. Call me a geek, but our ability to finally illuminate the ways in which these plant molecules enhance our health gets me so excited!

Plant and Fungal Molecules That Produce Hormetic Effects on Health and Longevity in Model Organisms and Humans

Compound	Source	Mechanism	Major Finding
Berberine	Chinese goldthread, dietary supplement	Autophagy↑	Life span↑ in flies; improvement of T2DM markers in humans
Curcumin	Turmeric spice, dietary supplement	Autophagy↑	Life span↑ in fruit flies (but failed to affect life span in mice); inflammation↓, hypertension↓, and ROS↓ in humans
Caffeine	Coffee	AMPK↑, mTOR↓, autophagy↑	Life span↑ in nematodes; CVD↓, cognitive impairment↓, and mortality↓ in humans
EGCG	Green tea, dietary supplement	SIRT1↑, FOXO↑, autophagy↑, Nrf2↑	Life span↑ in rats; cardiovascular disease↓, cancer↓, and neuroprotection↑ in humans
Emodin	Rhubarb and Chinese herbs	Sir2.1↑, AMPK↑	Life span↑ in nematodes; insulin sensitivity↑ in mice
Fisetin	Strawberry, apple, persimmon, grape, onion, and cucumber	DAF-16/FOXO↑, ROS↓, CRP↓	Life span↑ in nematodes; inflammation↓ in humans

Compound	Source	Mechanism	Major Finding
Glucosamine	Dietary supplement	AMPK↑, autophagy↑	Life span↑ in nematodes and mice; mortality↓ in humans
Polyphenols	Coffee	AMPK↑, mTOR↓, autophagy↑	CVD↓, cognitive impairment↓, and mortality↓ in humans
Polysaccharides	The mushrooms cordyceps and reishi	Prebiotic, intestinal integrity↑	Obesity↓, inflammation↓, diabetes↓ in HFD-fed mice
Quercetin	Vegetables such as apples and onions, dietary supplement	AMPK↑, autophagy↑, senescence↓	Life span↑ in mice; hypertension↓ in humans
Resveratrol	Red wine, dietary supplement	IGF-1↓, AMPK↑, PGC-1α↑, autophagy↑	Life span↑ in HFD-fed mice; improved markers for Alzheimer's disease, cancer, CVD, T2DM in humans
Spermidine	Soybeans, natto, fungi	Autophagy↑	Life span↑ in mice; mortality↓ in humans
Sulforaphane	Broccoli, Brussels sprouts, and other cruciferous vegetables	Nrf2↑, antioxidant enzymes↑	Neuroprotection↑ in rats

Source: Martel J, Ojcius DM, Ko YF, et al. "Hormetic Effects of Phytochemicals on Health and Longevity." *Trends Endocrinol Metab.* 2019 Jun;30(6):335–46.

Abbreviations: AMPK, adenosine-monophosphate-activated protein kinase; CRP, C-reactive protein; CVD, cardiovascular disease; EGCG, epigallocatechin gallate; FOXO, forkhead box O; HFD, high-fat diet; IGF-1, insulin-like growth factor 1; mTOR, mammalian target of rapamycin; Nrf2, nuclear factor (erythroid-derived 2)-related factor 2; PGC-1α, peroxisome proliferator-activated receptor γ coactivator 1α; ROS, reactive oxygen species; SIRT1, sirtuin-1; Sir2.1, sirtuin-2.1; T2DM, type-2 diabetes mellitus.

One of the simplest ways to activate your longevity pathways is to include a rich variety of phytochemicals in your diet, especially the ones noted in the previous table along with a few others such as Himalayan Tartary buckwheat and urolithin A, which have been proven to work on our ancient healing and repair systems. They induce our cells to become more stress resilient and activate a whole set of pathways designed to protect our cells from disease and aging.

PROTEIN AND AGING: WHERE'S THE BEEF?

Among the biggest controversies in nutrition and in the field of aging research is protein. Some declare plant proteins to be the only safe proteins for health and longevity. Others suggest meat is the best source of protein to prevent aging and sarcopenia. Remember Emma Morano, the Italian woman who lived to be 117 years old, who was told by her doctor in her nineties to eat 150 grams of raw meat a day? She was dwindling, and clearly this worked for her. Beliefs, ideologies, and preferences aside, what does the science say about protein and healthy aging? What protein, how much protein, when do we need to eat protein?[36]

The key question is how do we build muscle, the currency of healthy aging, and prevent and reverse sarcopenia, while at the same time not overstimulating the mTOR pathway and preventing autophagy, essential to recycle, repair, and renewal? A low level of amino acids and sugars mimics starvation, which kicks in autophagy and our longevity pathways. That's a good thing. But too much of a good thing can be bad. If we have no or low levels of protein or inadequate levels of certain amino acids like leucine, in the long haul that will keep mTOR activity low, but we will waste away into frailty. It's the Goldilocks problem.

The good news is that many of the world's experts gathered to answer these questions. They formed the PROT-AGE Study Group,[37] and they reviewed evidence in the following five areas:

1. Protein needs for older people in good health
2. Protein needs for older people with specific acute or chronic diseases
3. The role of exercise along with dietary protein for recovering and maintaining muscle strength and function in older people
4. The practical aspects of providing dietary protein (i.e., the source and quality of dietary proteins, timing of protein intake, and ensuring enough calories from fat and carbohydrates so that dietary protein won't be turned into energy but turned into muscle)
5. The use of functional outcomes to assess the impact of age- and disease-related muscle loss and the effects of interventions

What do we know about protein and aging?

As people age, they lose muscle and bone and their immune systems decline in function, all systems dependent on high-quality protein. Their appetites decrease, they take medications that may impair nutrient absorption, and their ability to use available protein decreases because they are more likely to be insulin resistant. And they have to work to compensate for something called *anabolic resistance*, which requires more protein than a younger person needs to build muscle. They also have greater needs for protein because of increased inflammation and oxidative stress.

When the body is in a state of breakdown, it needs far more protein.

The typical recommendation for daily protein intake (or RDA, recommended dietary allowance) is 0.8 mg/kg per person, per day. This is the *minimum* necessary to prevent protein malnutrition, not the amount for optimal health or for the aging population or the very active. Remember, preservation of muscle mass and preventing sarcopenia are the keys to staying active, functional, and metabolically healthy as we age.

The best way to build muscle is to eat muscle.

What did the PROT-AGE experts find?

1. To maintain and regain muscle, people over sixty years old need more dietary protein than do younger people; they should consume an average daily intake in the range of 1.0 to 1.2 g/kg of body weight a day. If they exercise—which they should—they may need 1.5 to 2.0 g/kg of body weight a day. For a 70-kilogram (11-stone) person that is 70 to 84 grams of protein a day. If you are doing weight training and aerobic exercise, you may need 105 to 140 grams a day (see the table later in this chapter for grams of protein in common foods).

2. The per-meal *anabolic threshold* (the amount of protein that triggers muscle building) of dietary protein and amino acid intake is higher in older individuals (i.e., 25 to 40 g protein per meal, containing about 2.5 to 2.8 g leucine) compared to that in young adults. If you eat less than that, the protein is used for calories and energy rather than for making muscle. Leucine, found primarily in animal protein, is essential because it is required to start protein synthesis.

3. The protein source (animal or plant), timing of intake, and amino acid supplementation need to be considered when making recommendations for dietary protein intake by older adults. Plant proteins alone are inadequate and must be supplemented with branched-chain amino acids high in leucine to activate muscle synthesis, or you need to consume large amounts of processed plant protein powders to get enough of the key muscle-building amino acids.

What are the essential things to remember?

1. The average person needs 25 to 40 grams of high-quality protein per meal, depending on age, activity level, and illness. That's a lot more protein than many get.

2. The best timing of protein intake is within an hour or two after exercise.

3. The best protein for muscle synthesis is animal protein because it contains high levels of leucine and creatine, also needed for protein synthesis.

4. Whey protein is the best source of easily absorbable high-quality protein that's high in leucine and other key amino acids for muscle building. I like regeneratively raised or organic goat whey. It is better tolerated by most. A protein shake after a workout is a powerful muscle-building strategy.

5. If you are using plant proteins, it is important to supplement with leucine, branched-chain amino acids, creatine, and even phyto-nutrients such as urolithin A, all of which I use in my Healthy Aging Shake (see Chapter 14).

6. If you have poor kidney function, your protein requirements are lower, and you must work with your doctor to determine the right amount of protein for you.

The other important thing to understand about protein is that if you eat more than you need, the excess protein is simply used as calories and can be turned into sugar by your body (via something call *gluconeogenesis*). Also many people use collagen protein, which is rich in glycine, proline, and hydroxyproline, all needed to build connective tissue, but is lacking in tryptophan, which must be added to make a complete protein.

The best rule of thumb is to eat a palm-sized piece of animal protein (or the equivalent in grams of whey protein or plant proteins) at every meal. If you are a 5-foot-tall (1.5-metre), 100-pound (45-kg) woman, your needs are different from those of a 6-foot-6-inch (2-metre), 250-pound (113-kg) man. Combining plant and animal proteins can be a helpful way to reduce animal protein (if that's your preference) without sacrificing protein quality.

Many plant-based advocates suggest we can get all our protein from beans, grains, nuts, and seeds. This is problematic for two reasons: first, the low levels of leucine and inadequate amino acid profiles required for turning protein to muscle and preventing it from just being used for energy; second, the sheer volume you'd need to get the 25 to 40 grams per meal. You would have to eat 800 grams of brown rice (an impossible feat per meal), which has 1,296 calories, to equal 115 grams of chicken, with 271 calories. To meet your daily protein needs from beans, you would need to eat 400 grams, with 450 calories, at each meal. It's just basic math and biochemistry.

Protein Source (30 grams)	Amount	Calories
Red meat	115 grams	285
Chicken	115 grams	271
Fish (cod)	175 grams	140
Whey protein	30 grams (1–2 scoops)	120
Eggs	5 eggs	390
Beans (black) cooked	400 grams	450
Quinoa (cooked)	740 grams	888
Brown rice	800 grams	1,296
Whole wheat bread	8.3 slices	573
Almonds	160 grams	942
Walnuts	300 grams	1,308
Pumpkin seeds	300 grams	713
Chia seeds	120 grams	600

Bottom line: Eat high-quality protein daily to meet your needs based on age, health concerns, and activity level, ideally 1.2 to 1.5 grams per kilogram per day if you are active (which you should be). Combine plant and animal proteins to improve overall protein quality. Add branched-chain amino acids and creatine for building muscle. Take a 12- to 16-hour break from eating each day (practice time-restricted eating) to allow mTOR to quiet down and induce autophagy. Add exercise and strength training, and voilà, you have a muscle-building longevity plan.

Chapter 8

Moving for Longevity

Those who think they have not time for bodily exercise will sooner or later have to find time for illness.

—EDWARD STANLEY, EARL OF DERBY

The simple rule of exercise is this: You have to move, or you won't! A cartoon I use in my lectures shows a doctor and a patient, and the caption reads, "Do you want to exercise an hour a day or be dead 24 hours a day?" It is not far from the truth. Exercise automatically improves all the hallmarks and root causes of aging. It improves blood sugar control and insulin sensitivity; helps control weight; and reduces the risk of heart disease, high blood pressure, and high cholesterol. It improves mood and motivation and cognitive function. It prevents dementia by increasing brain-derived neurotrophic factor (BDNF), a compound that increases neuroplasticity and builds new brain cells. It obviously improves muscle strength and bone health, preventing the ravages of frailty that we often see with biological aging and a sedentary lifestyle. Exercise also reduces the risk of many cancers, such as colon, breast, uterine, and lung. It improves sleep. And if your libido is low or sexual function is waning, it helps with that, too, by boosting testosterone in men and women. Maybe that will get you moving!

EXERCISE: THE POWER OF MOVEMENT

Exercise (the right dose, type, and frequency) optimizes all the biological systems. It improves the function and health of your microbiome, enhances immune function, boosts the number and function of mitochondria, and balances blood sugar and insulin, adrenal, thyroid, and sex hormones. It also boosts detoxification, blood circulation, and lymphatic flow. Looking at the hallmarks of aging, it increases telomere length, reduces inflammation, improves mitochondrial health, beneficially impacts the nutrient-sensing pathways, and reverses harmful epigenetic changes that occur as we age.

For example, when you deplete energy in your muscles and organs via exercise, AMPK is activated, improving insulin sensitivity (see "Hallmark 1" in Chapter 4). That, in turn, inhibits mTOR, resulting in autophagy and cellular cleanup. Exercise also activates the key longevity sirtuin pathway to induce DNA repair and reduce inflammation. It causes a slight bump in oxidative stress, which then triggers the activation of your antioxidant enzymes. The science is clear now on how exercise has so many health and longevity benefits.[1]

And it doesn't take much.[2] Fewer than 23 percent of Americans meet the recommended amount of exercise (150 minutes of moderate exercise or 75 minutes of vigorous exercise per week). But even something as simple as walking 10 minutes per day can add years to your life.[3] Walking is great, but more vigorous activity for about 75 to 150 minutes a week is better. Add in three to four days of strength training with bands, weights, or body-weight exercises, including squats, push-ups, shoulder presses, chest presses, and planks.

EXERCISE, MOVEMENT, AND LONGEVITY

Combined with the right diet, exercise is the most powerful tool for staying healthy and extending your life. My mother used to say that whenever she had the urge to exercise, she would lie down until it went away. Sadly, not the best strategy. She ended up frail and disabled for the last decade of her life. I bought her a book called *Growing Old Is Not for Sissies,* which featured stories of extraordinary athleticism in people in their seventies to nineties. She wasn't too happy about the gift. Centenarians now compete in track and field! Personally, my plan is to win the eighty-and-over tennis championship! For me health and healthy aging means I can wake up and do whatever it is I want that day. Take a walk, climb a mountain, go skiing, or skydive! In Ikaria I had trouble keeping up with Alkea, an eighty-seven-year-old woman who nimbly climbed up and down her mountainside terraces like a mountain goat as she tended her garden.

Exercise is the key to unlocking the body's regenerative and reparative systems. It activates all the longevity switches (through hormesis), increases the body's antioxidant systems, and improves cognitive function and mood. Exercise supports a healthy and diverse microbiome,[4] reduces chronic inflammation,[5] supports mitochondrial health and biogenesis,[6] helps balance hormones[7] and lowers cortisol (the stress hormone), keeps your body strong as you age,[8] supports detoxification, circulation, and lymphatic flow, and increases overall happiness and satisfaction with life.[9] It even makes your sex life better!

The research on exercise and longevity is indisputable. Exercise protects your telomeres,[10] increases telomere length, optimizes the beneficial metabolic effects of AMPK,[11] activates sirtuins,[12] and improves longevity and health span overall.[13] Exercise improves heart and cardiovascular health, decreases the risk of heart disease, and improves the outcomes of those with heart disease.[14] Exercise has been proven to prevent certain types of cancer, improves outcomes during treatment, and also prevents recurrence of cancer.[15] It is a powerful treatment for diabetes, improves blood sugar, and is key to improving insulin sensitivity.[16] And most important, it helps you build and improve muscle function and mass. Remember all the dangers of muscle loss and sarcopenia? The right exercise plus the right types and amounts of protein are your ticket to a long, healthy life.[17] I don't like the gym or traditional exercise but love to play. Go for a hike or a bike ride, play sports, or just take a 30-minute walk after dinner.

If you want to age well, live long, and be functional, regular exercise is not optional. Want to live to be 120 or more? Improve your health span? Reduce your risk for chronic diseases? Or simply *feel* better and happier? All of the above? Move.

Chapter 9

Optimizing Your Lifestyle for Longevity: Beyond Diet and Exercise

No matter how much it gets abused, the body can restore balance. The first rule is to stop interfering with nature.

—DEEPAK CHOPRA

As you have learned, it is your individual exposome washing over your genes that determines your health. Your genes are not your destiny. They load the gun, but your environment pulls the trigger. This is good news. Your daily behaviors are the single biggest factor in your health.

When I visited Sardinia and Ikaria, so many of the oldest residents were engaged in daily habits that have kept them strong, vibrant, and alive. They moved regularly, gardening and hiking up and down the rugged mountains, lived with little stress, prioritized sleep and naps, and had a deep sense of purpose and meaning. These are the types of practices you can start implementing today, but they require a little more intention because they are not the automatic defaults of our environment. Once you have built the foundation of a health-promoting longevity lifestyle, including the right diet and exercise, rest, stress management, sleep, and finding your community and purpose, you may want to include some other practices such as hormesis (see Chapter 10) and advanced longevity innovations (see Chapter 11) to boost your longevity pathways and stave off the hallmarks of aging.

Finding the tools and resources needed to live a long and healthy life can be daunting. I have compiled a list of the best resources for optimizing your lifestyle, including diet, exercise, stress management, sleep, supplements, and everything you need to track your biomarkers and health metrics. It is all at youngforeverbook.com/resources.

HEALING OUR MINDS, HEARTS, AND SPIRIT: THE ANTIDOTE TO THE DANGERS OF CHRONIC STRESS

Many of us tend to put self-care last on our list of to-dos (I certainly have for much of my life, to the detriment of my own health). Work, family, friends, and the needs of others often come first. Nourishing our spirit and mental health is usually an afterthought or not a thought at all. In places like the Blue Zones, the power of rest and community is central to life. But our fast-paced society — full calendars, many extracurricular activities, building careers, raising families, and taking work home — has made self-care and mental health low priorities. The truth is you cannot live a healthy, happy, fulfilled, and long life while neglecting to nourish your mind and spirit.

It might be hard to imagine, but your thoughts, feelings, beliefs, grief, joy, sadness, love, and anger are all transmuted into biological signals that change your gene expression, impacting your immune function, hormones, microbiome, neurotransmitters, neuroplasticity, mitochondria, and more. Getting your mind and mindset right has profound health benefits. Study after study has shown, for example, how repressed anger can predict who gets breast cancer and other cancers. If your emotions are inflamed, so is your biology. Caroline Myss, an author and medical intuitive, says that your "biography becomes your biology." Neuroscientist Candace Pert wrote about the "molecules of emotion," based on her groundbreaking research at the National Institutes of Health, and established the field of psychoneuroimmunology.

Everyone must find their own way to heal their mind, heart, and spirit. Nourishing your spirit includes cultivating a positive mindset (optimists live longer even if they are wrong!), developing self-love and self-worth, prioritizing self-care, cultivating community and meaningful relationships, practicing healthy stress-management techniques, finding support, and practicing religion or spirituality if that speaks to you.

Nourishing your spirit is especially tough for the natural givers, or "care-a-lots"—those who dedicate their lives to helping others. The best and only sustainable way to help others is to prioritize your own spirit. By making sure your cup is filled, you'll be able to fill others' cups, ten times over.

There is a mountain of empirical evidence to show that self-care, mindset, and community help improve all factors of health and longevity. Practicing self-compassion can significantly help people improve their health behaviors, like quitting smoking, exercising, eating healthier or overcoming eating disorders, practicing self-care, and improving overall well-being.[1] Self-compassion is also associated with improving physical symptoms,[2] mental health outcomes, glycemic control in patients with diabetes,[3] and resiliency against certain cancers as well as improved mental health in those with cancer.[4]

Social connections, community, and strong relationships have been associated with increased life span, improved mental health, and improved physical markers such as blood pressure, waist circumference, body mass index, and inflammation.[5]

Mindset, another feature of spiritual health, is also scientifically important. Research shows that people who ruminate over negative thoughts tend to have decreased life spans and poorer physical and mental health.[6] Those who focus on positive thoughts and future goals and rewards have better well-being and physical health.[7]

Having a sense of purpose is associated with overall well-being, improved physical and cognitive health, reduced depressive symptoms, and slower aging.[8] In fact, psychological well-being is even associated with increased telomere length and slower telomere attrition,[9] whereas chronic stress is associated with decreased telomere length, accelerated cellular aging, and increased oxidative stress.[10]

So, taking care of yourself, practicing self-love and self-compassion, working on a growth mindset, building relationships and community, and having a sense of purpose are crucial to living a fulfilling, long, healthy life. Prioritizing self-care and making time for reflection, relaxation, and mindfulness can support healthy hormone levels. Studies have shown that interventions like meditation and mindfulness can significantly lower cortisol levels.[11] So, make sure you're taking time for you.

OPTIMIZING SLEEP FOR LONGEVITY

When I was a medical student and resident, sleep was considered optional. Delivering 500 babies and working in the emergency department for overnight shifts fried my nervous system. I learned firsthand the dangers of sleep deprivation. Sleep, while it may seem superfluous, is essential to our health and longevity. The notion of "I will sleep when I am dead" may cause you an early death. It affects every aspect of our health, including our metabolism, weight, mood, and cognitive function.

Over the last 100 years the average sleep has declined by an hour or two. Seventy million Americans suffer from sleep problems.[12] Lack of sleep not only impairs our ability to concentrate and causes trouble learning, decreased attention to detail, and increased risk of motor vehicle accidents; research suggests that regularly sleeping for less than 7 hours a night has negative effects on the cardiovascular, endocrine, immune, and nervous systems. Side effects of sleep deprivation can include obesity, diabetes, heart disease, high blood pressure, anxiety, depression, dementia, alcohol abuse, stroke, and increased risk of developing some types of cancer.

Sleep is essential for healing and repair and cellular cleanup and longevity.[13] A newly discovered brain–cleaning system called the *glymphatic system* is essentially the lymph system of the brain and necessary for cleaning up all the metabolic waste that accumulates every day. Your muscles, organs, and brain need to repair each day. Your hormones and circadian rhythms must be in balance for health and longevity, and sleep is critical to maintaining that balance. If you sleep less than 7 hours a night, your risk of death increases by 24 percent. If you want to understand the importance of sleep, you must read Matthew Walker's book, *Why We Sleep.*

MEANING AND PURPOSE

Meaning makes a great many things endurable—perhaps everything. Through the creation of meaning . . . a new cosmos arises.

—C. G. JUNG

In places like the Blue Zones, people seem to understand their place and purpose in the community in which they live. There is an embedded sense of meaning and purpose that guides their lives. Many of us in this chaotic, hurried, often disconnected world struggle to find our way. But it is an essential ingredient for health.

Dr Robert Butler, the first director of the National Institute on Aging, performed a study that looked at having a sense of purpose and life expectancy. He found that people who have a clear sense of purpose, a reason to get up in the morning, lived up to seven years longer than those who didn't have a clear purpose. In another study of 7,000 adults, published in the *Journal of the American Medical Association,* those who had the lowest life purpose scores were twice as likely to die as those with the highest scores.[14]

How can you find your purpose? Richard Leider, who authored *The Power of Purpose,* provides a useful framework for identifying your purpose, your why. He says that your gifts plus your passions and values equals your purpose. Dig deep to find what you love and follow that road. It is different for each of us, but it is as essential as eating well and exercising for your longevity. It is no accident that the risk of death goes way up after retirement—and it's not just because of chronological age.

The science of altruism shows that being part of something bigger, helping others, and being of service is one of the most powerful roads to meaning and happiness. I remember in the aftermath of the 2010 Haiti earthquake, working 20 hours a day serving the wounded in the main hospital in Port-au-Prince, barely eating, facing the worst trauma and death and loss I had ever seen, I felt grateful to be of service to others, doing something meaningful and not focused on myself.

The foundations of health and longevity—diet, exercise, sleep, learning to manage stress and rest our nervous system, building meaningful relationships and community, and finding purpose and meaning in your life—are available to all of us at little or no extra cost in our lives. Just getting these habits and practices embedded in your daily life will make profound changes in your health and extend your life span.

For those of you who want to dive deeper, to explore additional powerful and novel strategies to reverse aging and live a longer, more vibrant life, for those who want to join me in reaching 120 years old in good health, you may want to take advantage of advanced innovations such as hormesis and regenerative medicine, which are covered in the next two chapters.

Chapter 10

Hormesis: Activating Healing and Repair Mechanisms

All things are poisons and nothing is without poison; only the dose permits something not to be poisonous.
— PARACELSUS, SIXTEENTH-CENTURY SWISS CHEMIST

The body is miraculously designed, containing within a profound set of innate healing mechanisms to keep us healthy and alive. Those healing systems are degraded by our modern diet, environment, and lifestyle, but science is discovering how to activate them. One of the keys to health and longevity is the simple principle that what doesn't kill you makes you stronger. When your system is stressed a little but not too much, it responds by becoming stronger and more resilient.

Think exercise. You stress your system by running fast or lifting weights, tearing your muscles, and in the healing process you become stronger. But overexercising can lead to injury. Similarly, a little cold stress and you activate healing; too much, you die of hypothermia. A little overheating repairs damaged proteins and boosts your immune system; too much, you die of heat stroke. The stress of caloric restriction consistently extends life in animal models by a third, or the equivalent of living to 120 years old. You can't eat so few calories that you will die, but a little starvation activates longevity pathways.

This phenomenon is called *hormesis*. Think of it as small doses of adversity or abundance that kick your body into high gear to protect itself. Hormesis may just be a big key to keeping us healthy and living a long, long time without disease or frailty.

The world of biohacking (essentially the layperson's version of functional medicine) incorporates many hormetic strategies:

- Time-restricted eating and fasting
- High-intensity interval training and strength training
- Cold plunges and saunas
- Breath work, hypoxia (low oxygen states)
- Hyperbaric oxygen therapy
- Ozone therapy
- Light therapy
- Phytochemicals

Even intellectual challenges—learning a new language or doing crossword puzzles—are examples of hormesis. These strategies produce effects by turning on a series of healing systems that activate DNA repair, cool off inflammation, increase your body's antioxidant systems, stimulate stem cell production, increase brain neuroplasticity, improve protein function, enhance detoxification, stimulate mitochondrial function and energy production, increase insulin sensitivity, and improve gene expression—all things necessary to prevent and reverse disease and extend healthy life span. Think of them as little stressors that make you more stress-resilient and metabolically flexible and help you adapt and survive.

Let's briefly explore the most powerful hormetic strategies for longevity. Each of these can be incorporated into your life. Some are simple, free, or inexpensive, and others are more expensive or require medical care.

CALORIE RESTRICTION

In Part I, you learned that calorie restriction activates the longevity switches to clean up and repair the body (autophagy and DNA repair).

In fact, in studies, the only thing that predictably extended life in animal models was eating a third fewer calories.[1] A deficit of calories also reverses insulin resistance, cools off inflammation, optimizes mitochondrial energy production, increases muscle mass, lowers fat mass, activates antioxidant systems, boosts stem cell production, and more.

The holy grail of aging science is hacking calorie restriction. Let's face it. If you eat a third fewer calories, you will be hungry, skinny, tired, and frail. You might live longer but you will be hangry all the time! I once met a man from the Calorie Restriction Society committed to living longer by eating less. I asked him what he ate for breakfast. His answer? Five pounds of celery. Not much fun.

Science is hard at work experimenting with diet, supplements, and medications that mimic caloric restriction without the pain and suffering. The good news is that many approaches are being explored that won't have you eating 5 pounds (2.3 kg) of celery a day. While the story is still being told, there seem to be many ways to mimic starvation without starving.

Fasting has become in vogue, and for good reason. Taking a break from eating for 12, 14, or 16 hours a day is the best way to activate autophagy through the nutrient-sensing pathways, including insulin signaling, mTOR, sirtuins, and AMPK. This is typically called *time-restricted eating.* Everyone should take a 12-hour break between dinner and breakfast; after all, it is called "break fast." Eat dinner at 6 p.m. and breakfast at 8 a.m., and you have a 14-hour fast. Extend breakfast to 10 a.m., and that's a 16-hour fast. Not so hard.

Another strategy being researched is the three- or seven-day water fast, known as *intermittent fasting,* once a month, or longer as a treatment for diabetes or obesity. Or a 24- to 36-hour fast weekly. Fasting-mimicking diets designed by the longevity researcher Valter Longo provide about 800 calories a day for five-day cycles repeated monthly or quarterly. Lastly, ketogenic diets (more than 70 percent fat and less than 5 percent carbohydrates) also mimic starvation and switch the body from running on carbohydrates to running on fat. It is likely best to cycle in and out of a ketogenic diet following our evolutionary pattern of alternating between periods of starvation and abundance. The key is to give your body a break from eating on a regular basis.

Certain plant compounds may mimic caloric restriction and lead to *xenohormesis,* activating autophagy. Some of these include the polyphenols in coffee; oleuropein, found in extra virgin olive oil; resveratrol, found in red grape skin and Japanese knotweed; sirtuin activating compounds, or STACs, such as fisetin from strawberries; spermidine (yes, it comes from where you think!); catechins, found in green tea; curcumin, found in turmeric; berberine; and a gut metabolite of pomegranate called urolithin A. Medications such as metformin and rapamycin may also exert their benefits in part by mimicking calorie restriction.

HEAT THERAPY: TURNING UP THE TEMPERATURE

Could the longevity benefits of being Finnish have something to do with the fact that there are enough saunas for every Finn to be in a sauna at the same time?[2] Scientists rigorously looked at the risk of death and cardiac events in more than 2,000 Finnish sauna users over 20 years. Since nearly everyone in Finland uses saunas at least once a week, that was the control group. The average temperature in the saunas was 78 degrees Celsius. Those who used a sauna two to three times a week had a 24 percent lower risk of death; and the hard-core users, who went four to seven times a week, had a 40 percent reduction in death compared to those who went for just one session a week.[3] Spending about 20 minutes versus 10 minutes in the sauna gives you a 52 percent lower risk of cardiac death.

Just how does a sauna, steam, hot bath, hot springs, or hot yoga prevent death and extend life span?

Anyone who has been in a sauna knows how you feel after. Invigorated, alert, energized, clear-headed, with a better mood, less stress, and less pain. Your heart rate and breathing and blood pressure rise as you sweat, just like they do when you exercise, but without moving. How do these benefits occur? Heat therapy works by increasing the production of heat shock proteins (HSPs). As we learned earlier, deformed and damaged proteins drive the aging process and need to be repaired or digested and cleaned up to be made into new proteins. Altered and damaged proteins are one of the hallmarks of aging.

Proteins are molecules that depend on their shape to function. Protein damage can manifest in malformed or unfolded proteins. HSPs help the proteins refold or, if they are too damaged, break them down and recycle them so damaged proteins don't accumulate. HSPs activate our internal antioxidant and repair systems. They prevent damage to proteins from oxidative stress and reduce AGEs, the advanced glycation end products formed from too much sugar binding to proteins and creating inflammation bombs.

Heat therapy also improves cardiovascular fitness, heart rate variability (a measure of the health of your autonomic nervous system and stress resiliency), insulin sensitivity, and blood sugar and blood pressure levels. Heat also increases endorphins for a natural high, reduces stress hormones, and improves sleep. It helps with depression, weight loss, and detoxification of toxic chemicals and metals. Amyloid is one of the dysfunctional proteins involved in Alzheimer's, and sauna therapy four times a week reduces the risk of dementia and Alzheimer's by 66 percent.[4] Heat therapy also boosts growth hormone, needed for repairing and rebuilding your tissues, joints, skin, and hair. Two 15-minute dry sauna sessions a day increase growth hormone release by 500 percent. Saunas also help your immune system fight infections and cancer and reduce inflammation.

Any type of heat therapy works, including saunas, infrared saunas, steams, hot baths, hot springs, and even hot yoga! Finding a way— even just a hot bath—to regularly boost your temperature is an easy, cheap, and rejuvenating strategy to improve your health span and address the root causes of aging.

COLD THERAPY: COOLING OFF FOR LONGEVITY

Two thousand years ago, Seneca, the famous Stoic philosopher, described himself as a cold-water enthusiast who inaugurated the first of every year with a plunge into the Virgo aqueduct. Thomas Jefferson used a cold foot bath every morning for six decades and died at the ripe old age of eighty-three. Hippocrates also extolled the virtues of cold plunges. Wim Hof, the Dutch motivational speaker and extreme athlete, has popularized them to improve your mood and health and has taught many to climb snowy mountains with just shorts on. Many traditional practices of the Finns and others included both the sauna and the ice plunge. Athletes regularly soak in ice baths to reduce pain and inflammation and improve recovery times. Staying in too long will result in hypothermia and death, but just the right temperature for the right amount of time can have profound health benefits, including boosting endorphins, strengthening our immune system and lowering inflammation, boosting metabolism and weight loss, improving circulation, and stimulating the vagus nerve, which activates your body's deep relaxation response. It also increases focus, mental clarity, and the pleasure neurotransmitter dopamine. The special type of fat found between your shoulder blades ("brown fat") gets turned on, stimulating heat and energy production. I spent a month in a winter cabin in Vermont and started every day with an ice-cold shower. Didn't need that cup of coffee!

Science supports the benefits of cold therapy such as cold-water swimming, cold showers, cold plunges, and cryotherapy, which is available at centers around the country.[5] Regular use reduces fatigue, improves mood and memory, and results in pain relief from inflammatory diseases such as arthritis or fibromyalgia. It also shunts blood away from your skin, driving oxygen and nutrients to your internal organs. It's a great way to detoxify, especially if you do a sauna first, increasing overall circulation, followed by the ice plunge to quickly flush your lymph system, carrying old waste and debris from your body back to the liver to be processed. The risks are few unless you have a serious underlying health condition, but you can build up slowly, starting with warmer temperatures and short-duration treatments.

Starting the day with a 1- to 2-minute cold shower is easy. A bath does nicely for a cold plunge, and you can even add bags of ice. Many companies now make easy-to-use temperature-regulated cold plunges. Or you can just get a water trough for animals and fill it with ice and water! A 1- to 4-minute cold plunge a day can be a powerful hack to your health, well-being, and longevity.

EXERCISE: PUSHING YOURSELF TO GET STRONGER AND LIVE LONGER

The most well-understood example of hormesis is exercise. All types. Compared to couch-surfing Netflix, vigorous exercise and strength training create a stress on your systems—a good stress, as it turns out. The mechanisms by which exercise improves health and longevity have been deeply studied.[6] Pushing your cardiovascular system and your muscles to work harder stimulates a cascade of longevity benefits.

Two things are highly correlated with longevity:

1. **Good aerobic capacity, as measured by VO$_2$ max.** Low levels put you at risk for disease and early death. In fact, in comparing the highest to the lowest levels of fitness using VO$_2$ max, the highest fitness group reduced their risk of death by 70 percent, with the biggest benefits in going from being sedentary to moderate fitness.[7] That means you don't have to be an extreme athlete to get the benefits of exercise; just get moving. And tennis players tend to live seven years longer than average.

2. **Muscle mass and function.** As we've discussed, sarcopenia is the invisible killer. We must fight the entropy of age-related loss of muscle function and mass with resistance or weight-training exercise while eating adequate amounts of high-quality protein. If we don't build more muscle, we will waste away. Use it or lose it. I tried to

ignore the benefits of strength training for 60 years, thinking that my running, biking, tennis, and yoga were enough. But they were not, and now at sixty-three years old with very little effort (30 minutes three times a week), I have dramatically increased my muscle mass, agility, strength, and stability.

Bottom line: This is one of the most powerful hormetic, health-creating, life-extending strategies you can use, and it's available to everyone. Want to be healthy, live long, and prevent frailty and disability as you age? Get moving and lifting!

LIGHT THERAPY: ON THE SPECTRUM TOWARD LONGEVITY

You might have heard of the dangers of blue light at night or seen people wearing blue-blocker glasses to look at their blue-light-emitting screens. You might even have heard of people bathing in red light to improve energy, recover from exercise, and reduce pain and inflammation. Is there a relationship between the quality of our light exposure and our health and life span? Is there a way to hack light? Whole companies have birthed to protect you from blue light and provide ways to heal with red-light therapy. There are even special nighttime light bulbs you can use to replace your fluorescent or LED lighting, both of which have no red light.

We are light-detecting devices. Our skin, our eyes, and our brain all receive light that, in turn, regulates our circadian rhythm and many other biological processes. Our evolutionary exposures to light used to be very predictable. We were exposed to bright light, including blue light, in the morning and daytime and then darkness after sunset. The light bulb changed all that, and fluorescent and LED lights changed it even more. In *Lights Out: Sleep, Sugar, and Survival*, T.S. Wiley and Bent Formby chronicle the ill effects of the light bulb. They include not just sleep deprivation, but also higher rates of diabetes, heart disease, cancer, and depression. Light regulates our hormones and neurotransmitters, which influence our appetite, fertility, and mental and physical health. Constant light exposure tricks our body into an endless summer, the time when our evolutionary pathways require us to store fat for the winter and slow our metabolism.

There is quite a bit of science about how light affects us.[8] We have all heard of seasonal affective disorder (SAD) from lack of light in the winter, or that the happiest people live in sunnier climes—these have been proven true. Short exposures to blue light can help treat depression and circadian sleep disorders, but prolonged exposure decreases life span in animal models and increases the risk for cancers, obesity, diabetes, and psychiatric disorders.[9]

Red and near-infrared light, on the other hand, acts as a very mild form of stress that activates protective mechanisms in cells. When red light hits the skin and penetrates cells, it stimulates the mitochondria to make more energy in the form of ATP, our body's fuel.[10] This, in turn, increases the production of natural anti-inflammatories and antioxidants and speeds up healing. Long-wavelength infrared and red-light therapy can improve eyesight, cognitive ability, physical mobility, and skin aging. There is even a term for it: *photobiomodulation*.[11]

Companies such as Joovv and others make devices that allow you to use this technology at home for improving skin health, reducing pain and inflammation, and improving cellular energy production.

OZONE THERAPY: THE KING OF HORMESIS

When we hear ozone, we think of the atmospheric ozone layer and its harmful effects on humans. If you read the FDA website, it will scare you to death. Ozone will kill you. And yes, it will, if you breathe it into your lungs. But water is deadly, too, if you inhale it. It's called drowning. Or if you drink too much water, it can dilute your blood and result in seizures, coma, or death, as is seen in long-distance runners who overhydrate. Should we stop drinking water? Clearly not. As of this writing, more than 4,000 scientific papers on ozone therapy are in the National Library of Medicine. It has a long use in medical practice globally. And there is a large body of science pointing to its effects in addressing chronic disease and extending life.[12]

Personally, I have experienced its benefits and so have hundreds of my patients. When I was very sick with mold toxicity, autoimmunity with uncontrollable colitis, and severe cognitive dysfunction, essentially wasting away with a weight loss of 30 pounds (13 kg) because of a cytokine storm, ozone therapy reversed 80 percent of my symptoms after just a few treatments. It has become a staple of my personal longevity strategy.

What is ozone? Is it safe? How does it work? And how can it help us live healthier and longer? Ozone, a gas discovered in the midnineteenth century, is a molecule consisting of three atoms of oxygen (O_3). Ozone has well-known toxic effects on the respiratory tract when present in smog and inhaled. In medical use, however, the gas produced from medical-grade oxygen is administered in precise therapeutic doses, and never via inhalation. Ozone therapy is simple to implement, effective, and well tolerated and has no significant side effects.[13] A survey of 644 practitioners in Germany who performed 5,579,238 treatments in 348,775 patients found an incidence of side effects of 0.00006 per treatment.[14]

Ozone therapy has been used and extensively studied for many decades. It is delivered in a low concentration combined with oxygen (usually about 2 to 5 percent ozone and 95 to 98 percent oxygen, which is why it is often called oxygen-ozone therapy. It can be administered via various routes, including intravenously, intramuscularly, rectally, and topically. Used to treat infections, wounds, and multiple diseases, ozone's effectiveness has been well documented for acute and chronic infections, autoimmune disease, and arthritis.[15]

O_3 is a highly reactive molecule that acts initially as a pro-oxidant and is also the world's most potent germicide. A short-term burst of oxidation triggers a whole set of responses that makes us stronger and healthier. When administered, ozone produces downstream compounds called ozonides that kill microbes and viruses, modulate the immune system, reduce inflammation, improve red blood cell pliability, destroy free radicals, enhance mitochondrial function, produce more stem cells, enhance oxygenation of resting muscles, and reduce blood clotting.[16] It is a powerful antidote to inflammaging and oxidative stress.

Medical oxygen-ozone therapy is a powerful hormetic therapy, activating several antiaging defense mechanisms in an easy-to-administer, safe, cost-effective, scalable treatment that has the potential to optimize our health and extend life.

HYPERBARIC OXYGEN THERAPY: OXYGEN UNDER PRESSURE

Every scuba diver knows about the decompression chamber, also known as the hyperbaric oxygen chamber, used to repressurize the body to prevent decompression sickness if they come up to the surface too fast. Athletes use hyperbaric oxygen therapy (HBOT) to heal injuries and recover faster. Medical uses include wound healing, treating resistant infections (bugs don't love oxygen), and, increasingly, treating hearing loss and aiding in stroke recovery, traumatic brain injury, chronic fatigue, and even dementia and Parkinson's. Could it extend life? Turns out it just might.

The treatment consists of "diving" down to what is the equivalent of more than 1 atmosphere below the surface of the ocean in a 100 percent oxygen environment. Being the equivalent of more than 33 feet/10 meters (1 atm, or atmosphere) to 66 feet/20 meters under the ocean (2 atm) in a fully oxygenated environment (room air is only 21 percent oxygen) is a hormetic stress to the body. Pure oxygen is toxic at high doses when administered for too long. But given at the right dose for the right duration under pressure, it kicks your system into healing mode and boosts longevity.

Scientists from Tel Aviv University treated thirty people over sixty-four years old with sixty sessions over ninety days in a chamber at 2 atm in a 100 percent oxygen environment.[17] They found that HBOT can get rid of zombie cells and lengthen telomeres better than any other lifestyle or medical intervention. They literally reversed the biological age of these participants in only three months. That is an impressive result for a safe, well-established medical treatment. HBOT also works to enhance health and extend life through other established mechanisms, such as increasing new blood vessel growth (good for the aging brain and heart) and mitochondria production. It also increases stem cell activity and activates sirtuins,[18] which improves nutrient sensing.

Soon this therapy may not just be for scuba divers, athletes, and those with difficult-to-treat wounds. It may prove to be a health-maintenance longevity strategy. While the "dose" of 2 atm used in this study requires a medical-grade chamber, lower doses may help, but more research is needed. Low-dose chambers can be safely used at home. Higher-dose at-home chambers are also now available. This is a low-risk strategy for longevity pioneers!

HYPOXIA: STARVING FOR AIR STIMULATES LONGEVITY PATHWAYS

Tibet, where people live at high altitudes in hypoxic or low-oxygen states, has an unusually high percentage of centenarians despite stressful living conditions.[19] The high mountain region of Vilcabamba, known as the valley of longevity in Ecuador, is also home to many long-lived humans, with people routinely living into their nineties and 100s. Worms in a lab deprived of oxygen live longer. Wild animals routinely exposed to low-oxygen states, such as the naked mole rat and bowhead whale, also live longer.[20]

Could low-oxygen states trigger longevity pathways? Just as high-pressure, high-oxygen states can trigger those pathways, so can low-pressure, low-oxygen states.

The body has a miraculously organized system to deal with all sorts of life stresses. These little stresses activate a cascade of downstream mechanisms designed to keep you alive. The stress of low oxygen triggers the production of a transcription factor (something that controls which genes are turned on or off) called *hypoxia inducible factor* that regulates more than 100 genes.[21] Short bursts of low-oxygen states can trigger an adaptive hormetic response, whereas prolonged hypoxia may accelerate aging, which is what happens with obstructive sleep apnea.

The low-oxygen states have their impact much in the way all stresses do—by triggering changes in the function of sirtuins, AMPK, and mTOR. They also lower inflammation and improve insulin sensitivity. Low-oxygen states also increase the production of stem cells and the formation of new blood vessels to help the body get more oxygen.

While it might be hard to climb to 10,000 feet every day and hang out, there are now devices that can simulate low- and high-oxygen states, equivalent to ascending Mount Everest for a few minutes then dropping down to sea level or even a higher oxygen state. This intermittent hypoxia-hyperoxia seems to trigger many beneficial effects, including improved blood sugar control[22] and cognitive function in dementia patients[23] and improved overall mitochondrial health. Low-oxygen states lead to the death of old mitochondria and stimulate the production of new and healthier mitochondria. All good things if you want to have energy and live a long time.

One such device is called the Cellgym, where a tight-fitting face mask is applied, and the machine puts you through four cycles of hypoxia with only 12 percent oxygen for 5 minutes followed by 3 minutes of hyperoxia, or high oxygen concentration, at 33 percent oxygen.

Other, simpler techniques can replicate some of the benefits, including ancient forms of breath work such as pranayama[24] or newer versions popularized by the Ice Man, Wim Hof, who recommends breath practice and cold plunges as a way of enhancing health, immunity, and overall well-being. I'll explain these and other hypoxia hacks in Part III: The Young Forever Program.

One of the key strategies to prevent disease, create health, and extend life is hormesis. These little stresses help our body activate ancient healing and survival mechanisms.

Clearly, it is a full-time job to incorporate all these strategies into your life, but I have learned to slowly incorporate many of these into my daily routine. Your week might look like this: Start with a 12- to 16-hour overnight fast daily. Incorporate into your diet phytochemicals (see Chapter 7), known to activate longevity pathways, including those in strawberries, turmeric, broccoli, green tea, pomegranate, Himalayan Tartary buckwheat, and mushrooms. Take a 2-minute cold shower or a cold plunge every morning, followed by short bursts of sprinting three or four times a week. Do strength training for 20 to 30 minutes three times a week. Add a sauna or steam as often as you can. Get blue-blocker glasses for the evening and replace your LED and fluorescent light bulbs with smart bulbs that adjust the light spectrum for the time of day, full spectrum in the day and red light for nighttime. Try a home red-light-therapy device. Explore intravenous ozone therapy or get an inexpensive home unit for rectal ozone therapy. Consider a course of hyperbaric oxygen therapy or try a Cellgym if there is one in your area or a low-oxygen exercise mask, which are available for $50 (£42). These tools are safe and available to us now, and they can provide a host of health and longevity benefits.

Chapter 11

Advanced Longevity Innovations

We cannot solve our problems with the same thinking we used when we created them.

—ALBERT EINSTEIN

The paradigm shift—the reframing of disease as an inevitable part of getting older to aging as a treatable disease—is driving billions of dollars of investment and research that will transform the landscape of health and longevity. Advances in medical science, functional medicine, the microbiome, wearable and implantable biotrackers, quantum computing, machine learning, and artificial intelligence are heralding a new era in medicine. We are deep in the shift from reductionist disease-based medicine to a systems-based ecological understanding of health and disease. It is propelling medicine toward a future that allows us to treat disease and reverse biological aging using both nature's intelligence and our body's own to repair, heal, and renew.

In this chapter we will explore exciting new advances that some longevity enthusiasts are using to help them optimize their health and increase their chance of living to well over 100 years old in good health. These are not affordable for most of us today, but like all other technologies, they will improve and prices will come down exponentially. My first computer cost \$3,500 (£3,000) and had a 4-megabyte hard drive and 1 megabyte of RAM. That same amount of storage today costs pennies.

Traditional medicine employs anti-inflammatories, beta-blockers, ACE inhibitors. These inhibiting, blocking, and anti-drugs can be useful, but they don't activate the body's own healing system, which is far more powerful than any medication. But in peeling back the layers of human biology, a whole new class of therapies is emerging that work very differently from traditional pharmacologic or surgical treatments. Rather than block or inhibit or interfere with some biological pathway, these therapies support and enhance the body's functioning. Think probiotics versus antibiotics. These therapies include NAD+ or its precursors, rapamycin (see "Hallmark 1" in Chapter 4), stem cells, exosomes, peptides, natural killer cells, plasmapheresis (a technique of cleaning the blood and removing inflammatory and aging molecules and proteins, much like *parabiosis,* where the blood of old mice is exchanged for the blood of young mice by linking up their circulatory systems and the old mice become younger), and ozone (covered in Chapter 10). These are all available now at the edges of health care. But there is more coming.

The futurist Ray Kurzweil talks about soon reaching *longevity escape velocity,* when advances in medicine and technology will allow us to outpace death. I am not sure I would vote for immortality. Death, in many ways, makes life more precious and meaningful. But it is intriguing. According to some scientists and futurists, we may be only ten to fifteen years away from achieving longevity escape velocity.

There are serious implications for extending life—and far more for immortality. How many people can the planet sustain? Will there be a net cost to society or a net benefit? In his paper in *Nature Aging* entitled "The Economic Value of Targeting Aging,"[1] Dr David Sinclair makes it clear: If we increase our collective health span and prevent or reverse chronic disease by addressing its root causes, it would create significant economic and social benefits. A healthy older population would unburden the health care system and dramatically reduce the nearly $4 trillion in health care expenditures in the United States, while increasing our life span. A healthy older population would continue to contribute to society. The social, political, and environmental implications of extending life are complex. They will require a reimagination of how we live and technological advances that will reduce the planetary burden of a larger population. In some ways, the limitations of our linear human mind cannot imagine this exponential change, or the ways that human ingenuity and creativity can — and have — exceeded what we had thought possible. In 1492 it was hard to imagine that the world was not flat, or that we would have access to all the world's knowledge in seconds on a device that would fit in the palm of our hand.

In 1894, the physicist Albert Michelson, who first measured the speed of light and won the Nobel Prize for physics in 1907, declared there was nothing more to discover in physics except a few decimal points. My grandfather was born in 1898 in a world without electricity, cars, planes, telephones, radio, television, or computers. We now take for granted air and space travel, and we carry a supercomputer in our pockets in the form of smartphones more powerful than the computers that landed man on the moon. Social media started with Facebook in 2004; now it is the main source of news, information, business, advertising, and communication for most of the world. The future of health care and the future of aging will look very different very soon.

We will soon see a world in which each of us will have our entire genome, microbiome, and metabolome (the sum total of all our biochemical pathways and reactions) mapped, a world of wearable or implantable devices that track thousands of our biomarkers in real time. All that data will be interpreted through artificial intelligence in the cloud and will allow us to identify subtle changes in our biology that precede disease by decades. We will be guided toward optimizing our diet, lifestyle, and habits to correct any early imbalances in real time.

Fantastical advances in medicine and technology are right around the corner, including 3D printing of organs that will make waiting for a new heart or kidney a quaint memory, and nanobots (microscopic robots) that will deliver precision medicines and treatments inside your body without side effects. Gene-editing tools such as CRISPR will allow us to rewrite our genome, to cure rare diseases, and to splice in genes that can optimize our biology. Yamanaka transcription factors, which we learned about in Chapter 1, will be inserted into our genome by a viral or gene-editing tool when we are in our twenties. As we age into our forties and notice a loss of muscle, gray hair, and wrinkles, and we have more aches and pains and feel the slow decline of our health and vitality, we will be able to use a molecular switch, like a remote control, for the Yamanaka factors, to reprogram our cells to their original embryonic state. This will turn back the biological clock, stop and reverse aging, eliminate gray hair and wrinkles, heal arthritis and chronic diseases, and rejuvenate our body back to its youthful vitality.[2] This *epigenetic rejuvenation* may seem like science fiction, but it is not too far down the scientific pike.

Gene reprogramming, gene editing, nanobots, and 3D organs are not available yet. But some promising treatments are available now that can help reverse diseases, optimize health, and potentially extend life. These treatments will soon become mainstream, but for longevity explorers they are available now in clinics around the world.

Regenerative medicine is a powerful new advance in longevity medicine that is available today in clinics in the United States and around the world. Mother Nature is, in fact, very smart. If you have injuries or damaged joints or tissues, her tool kit of stem cells, exosomes, peptides, and placental matrix is powerful in relieving pain; restoring mobility and function from even severe injuries, trauma, or degeneration; and reversing aging.

STEM CELLS: THE FOUNTAIN OF YOUTH

One of the key hallmarks of aging is the exhaustion of our stem cells. As we age, our stem cells age too, and their ability to regenerate tissues and cells, to repair and heal our bodies, declines. Emerging science suggests that intravenous infusions or injections into worn-out body parts like joints can rejuvenate the body.[3] The frailty of aging, manifested as a decline in muscle mass, endurance, energy, and organ function, may be reversed with stem cells. Think of them as cells that contain the memory of youth, that have the capacity to repair cells and regenerate tissues. They also secrete factors that regulate the immune system, reduce inflammation, and stimulate healing throughout the body. And they produce *exosomes,* little packets of healing factors that contain proteins, peptides, and microRNA (see the next section). Studies have shown that stem cell and exosome therapy significantly reduces the inflammation associated with aging while increasing energy and physical performance.[4]

The field of stem cell therapy is advancing fast. There are two major types of stem cells in the body: hemopoietic stem cells (HSCs), which come from bone marrow and help us replace our white and red blood cells; and mesenchymal stem cells (MSCs), which come from our tissues. HSCs can be harvested from bone marrow, and MSCs from fat cells.

Using our bodies' own stem cells can be effective, although this process is expensive and requires a painful procedure. Using umbilical or placental stem cells may be more effective because they are younger, and you can culture and harvest far more of them. These are obtained from umbilical cord blood or placental tissue (usually thrown away after birth)[5] and then grown or cultured in a lab. They can be injected intravenously for system healing or into specific body parts for localized repair and regeneration and will not be rejected by your immune system because of their unique immunoprotected nature. Stem cells can help renew the brain, heart, immune system, and mitochondria as well as increase testosterone and improve insulin sensitivity.

The United States has strict regulations that prohibit the harvesting and growing of stem cells. In other words, you cannot yet harvest your own stem cells and grow them in a lab to create a clinically meaningful dose to be injected into your blood, tissues, organs, or joints. Countries that allow the culturing of stem cells include Mexico, the Bahamas, Panama, Costa Rica, and others. The same is true for umbilical and placental stem cells. They can be grown in the United States but not administered in America. Much research remains to be done, but stem cell therapy will eventually become a routine intervention in medicine and the treatment of aging.

EXOSOMES: PACKETS OF YOUTH

What if you didn't need to harvest stem cells from your bone marrow or fat tissue (both painful medical procedures), or use expensive umbilical or placental stem cells to get the benefits of stem cell therapy? What if a treatment costing one-tenth the cost of stem cell therapy could be administered intravenously or into joints or tissues, give the same or nearly the same benefit, and have no side effects? Exosomes, little packets of growth factors, anti-inflammatory cytokines, lipids, proteins, DNA, and microRNA produced by stem cells, are emerging as an important therapeutic agent in medicine and regenerative medicine.[6] Exosomes have many functions, but they primarily act as messengers and communications systems between cells. They were first discovered in 1983 and are now known to have significant therapeutic benefits—to dramatically reduce inflammation, cross over the blood-brain barrier, and improve muscle and brain function. They also regulate the immune system, cellular cleanup and repair, and autophagy, and they play a role in treating autoimmune disease, obesity, and infectious disease. They can help repair and regenerate bone, cartilage, soft tissues, the heart, and the brain.[7] I used them to help cure my autoimmune disease—ulcerative colitis—and to heal my back after complications from back surgery. I also used them after I had COVID-19 and was struggling with fatigue, brain fog, and depression. The symptoms disappeared after only one treatment. While this may have been true just for me, exosomes have been effective for many of my patients in treating injury, autoimmunity, and chronic infections.

How do we produce exosomes for clinical use? Stem cells are harvested from placental tissue or amniotic fluid and cultured in a lab; then the exosomes are extracted, concentrated, and made available for treatment. Many clinics now offer this therapy for a variety of chronic conditions and as a longevity treatment. Exosomes can be easily given intravenously in multiple doses over time without any side effects.[8] While more research on their optimal use and effectiveness is needed, many aging biohackers routinely use exosomes to treat disease and enhance their health.

PEPTIDES: THE MAGICAL POWER OF THE BODY'S MINI-PROTEINS

If you are interested in regenerative or functional medicine, you may have heard of the power of peptides.[9] As we age the number and quality of peptides decline. What are they? What do they do? And how can they be used to treat disease, optimize health, and rejuvenate the body? We are all familiar with one peptide that has saved millions of lives: insulin! Peptides are mini-proteins made by the body to regulate nearly every biological function. More than 7,000 peptides are produced by the body—150 peptides are being researched for medical applications, and more than 80 peptides are already approved by the FDA for medical therapies.[10] Peptide therapies account for $70 billion (£60 billion) in sales worldwide.

Peptides are safe and easily synthesized in the lab. They can accelerate healing, boost hormone levels, improve immunity, fight infections, heal the gut, improve tissue repair, build muscle mass, decrease joint and muscle pain, enhance cognitive function and memory, optimize mitochondrial function, help reverse symptoms of sexual dysfunction, improve sleep quality, increase levels of energy, stamina, and strength, lower blood pressure, reduce signs of aging, and stimulate hair growth.[11] They are increasingly being used as a key therapeutic agent in traditional, functional, and regenerative medicine.[12] They are well tolerated and easily metabolized by the body. Since they are mini-proteins and would be digested by the gut if consumed orally, they are usually given by subcutaneous injection. Newer formulations include intranasal, sublingual (under the tongue), and implantable peptides.

Peptides are generally made from animal or plant protein sources such as eggs, milk, meat, soy, oats, flaxseed, hemp seed, and wheat. (Just more proof that food is medicine!) I have used them extensively in my practice and on myself. They have strengthened my immune function, helped my recovery from COVID-19, improved sleep, sexual function, and libido, and helped me heal from various injuries. I recently developed tendonitis in my shoulder, and with two injections of BPC-157 peptides, I was completely pain-free.

It is important to use the highest-quality peptides produced by compounding pharmacies that ensure the highest-quality manufacturing process and use pharmaceutical standards. They should be prescribed by a trained physician. Some peptides have become pharmaceuticals—such as semaglutide (Ozempic), used to treat diabetes and help with weight loss—and others are available from compounding pharmacies.

Here are a few promising peptide therapies:

- Thymosin alpha-1 (Zadaxin) helps the immune system combat immunological aging, autoimmune disease, and infections and is a powerful anti-inflammatory.
- BPC-157 activates growth factors and helps heal the gut and repair ligaments, tendons, and skin.
- Sermorelin and tesamorelin stimulate the body to produce growth hormone and improve muscle mass, mobilize stored fat for energy use, improve recovery from exercise, and improve skin health.
- MOTS-c, SS 31, and humanin are mitochondrial peptides that improve energy production as well as liver, muscle, and brain health.
- PT-141 (bremelanotide) stimulates the part of the brain that is responsible for sexual arousal and libido.
- Melanotan 1 helps improve skin and hair health, decreases appetite, and improves metabolism.
- GHK-Cu and GHK are anti-inflammatories that stimulate collagen creation.

NATURAL KILLER CELL THERAPY: MOBILIZING OUR ANTICANCER, INFECTION-FIGHTING CELLS

Many of us are walking around with low-grade chronic viral infections, tick-borne infections, and cancer cells, all of which our immune systems must manage. One of our body's main defenses is a special type of immune cell called the *natural killer cell*. These cells are exactly what they sound like, special forces that seek out and destroy infectious agents and cancer cells.

As we age, our natural killer cell function declines and cancer and infections increase. Technologies for harvesting and growing natural killer cells are emerging that will allow us to get a big dose of these powerful protective cells.[13] While not in widespread use, this emerging therapy will likely soon become a routine part of treating infections, cancer,[14] and aging itself.[15] I recently had my blood drawn and sent to a lab to culture my own natural killer cells; these were then infused back into my body to help me recover from Lyme disease and babesiosis, another tick-borne infection.

TRANSFER PLASMA EXCHANGE: CLEANING THE BLOOD

Studies show that when the circulation of an old mouse is connected to that of a young mouse, the old mouse becomes biologically younger. This is called *parabiosis*. The opposite is true, too—if you give a young mouse old blood, it ages rapidly. Is there a way to clean and rejuvenate your blood? Yes—through *transfer plasma exchange,* or *plasmapheresis*.

In your blood, you have red cells, white cells, and platelets swimming around in a sea of fluid known as *plasma* that contains thousands of proteins—proteins that become increasingly inflammatory as you age. Therapeutic plasma exchange removes your blood, separates the cells from the plasma, throws out the old inflammatory plasma, and replaces it with fresh albumin, the main protein in your blood. It has been effective in treating autoimmune diseases such as multiple sclerosis, myasthenia gravis, and Guillain-Barré syndrome, a paralytic neurological condition triggered by infections and vaccines. It has been shown to reduce cognitive decline in Alzheimer's by 66 percent.[16] It has also shown promise in treating long-haul COVID.[17] Much research is needed to assess its effects on aging, but it seems to work quickly, to be very safe, and to have profound long-lasting regenerative effects.

What has not been clear is this: Do factors in young blood make the old mice reverse aging? Or are there harmful blood-borne factors in old mice that cause rapid aging? A powerful study found that simply cleaning out the harmful factors in old blood using plasmapheresis was enough to reverse biological aging and rejuvenate old mice.[18] The study showed that a single plasma exchange created powerful rejuvenating effects. It enhanced muscle repair, reduced liver fat and scarring, and increased the formation of new memory cells in the brain. The process of cleaning the blood reset the mice's system, increased proteins that help with tissue repair and a healthy immune response, reducing inflammation and resulting in long-lasting changes in gene expression and molecular signaling that reverse aging. This might sound strange, but it is an FDA-approved treatment that could be an important tool in restoring health and resilience in an older population. It is a relatively simple, cost-effective, and safe procedure that may soon become a regular part of our health maintenance.

REGENERATIVE MEDICINE: TAKE THE BODY IN FOR REPAIRS

I have had many injuries that left me in chronic pain. I first had back surgery at thirty-two years old for a ruptured disc that left me with a paralyzed calf and a lifelong limp. For the last 30 years I have had chronic lower back pain that I managed with yoga and massage. I have bad arthritis and degenerative scoliosis in my lower back. Then at sixty I had another disc injury and another surgery that led to severe complications and bleeding into my spinal cord, which left me barely able to walk and in chronic pain. I then decided to try regenerative medicine with Dr Matt Cook from BioReset Medical, who radically transformed my pain and my life. I underwent a healing protocol that completely healed my body. He used exosome injections into my spinal canal to reduce inflammation and stimulate tissue repair. He also used injections of placental matrix, a complex mixture of anti-inflammatory and healing factors that holds significant promise in tissue and joint repair.[19] He injected healing factors—including exosomes, placental matrix, and peptides—in a procedure called hydro-dissection[20] to free up scarred fascia, nerves, and muscles and relieve pain. And he topped it off with injections of peptides and ozone. I am now pain-free and stronger than ever.

These therapies, collectively called *regenerative medicine,*[21] are increasingly being used to treat chronic pain and injury with great success. Placental matrix, for example, is rich in collagen, glycosaminoglycans, proteoglycans, and anti-inflammatory cytokines that promote repair of tissues and the growth of new blood vessels and reduce inflammation and scarring.

I also had a frozen shoulder for six months after I broke my arm. I couldn't lift my arm more than 30 degrees from the side of my body. Within 5 minutes of an injection of Prolozone, a mixture of 97 percent oxygen and 3 percent ozone, into my shoulder joint, I had full motion of my shoulder without any pain. Frozen shoulders often last for years, or forever, and need to be treated for months and months with painful physical therapy, or need traumatic manipulation under anesthesia, both barbaric. Prolozone can be injected into joints, muscles, and tendons to reduce inflammation and stimulate tissue repair.[22] I have patients with severe knee osteoarthritis who walked in on crutches and left the office dancing. It is very safe and inexpensive and can bring relief to many.

These therapies are not widely available yet but are becoming more and more available through regenerative medicine clinics. They will prove to be essential in the field of orthopedics and pain management.

*   *   *

You made it through the science of how our bodies work, how we age, and how diet, lifestyle, hormesis, and other innovations in longevity medicine can help us live better, healthier, and longer. Now we get to the practical application of all this science.

Next up: the Young Forever Program, a step-by-step road map to diagnose the imbalances in your system and to implement a radical change in your health.

PART III

THE YOUNG FOREVER PROGRAM

Chapter 12

The Young Forever Program: Overview

We are not proponents of a long life. We are proponents of a joyful life, and when you find yourself in joy, the longevity usually follows. We do not count the success of a life by its length; we count it by its joy.

—ABRAHAM (FROM CHRISTIANE NORTHRUP)

I plan to live to be 120, maybe even 180, in good health, savoring the miraculous gift of this life every day. That means staying active, sharp, strong, energetic, and engaged at every age. With the emerging research on longevity and the right mindset, I believe that's possible for all of us.

You can start turning back the clock today. Our simple daily habits dramatically impact the way we age, and the Young Forever Program will be your guide to preventing chronic illness, reversing your biological age, and living long and well. By focusing on health span as opposed to just life span, you can put more life in your years and more years in your life.

Longevity and aging research is accelerating at an exponential pace. More discoveries and strategies are emerging nearly every day. However, the foundational principles of preventing disease, creating health, and extending life are clear today. Biological aging is a treatable disease. The hallmarks of aging we've covered in *Young Forever* may be slightly modified as more research uncovers the mysteries of life and death, but they remain the framework for understanding *what* goes wrong and illuminating targets for treatment.

But the hallmarks of aging don't fully explore *why* they happen, the root causes of the deterioration we see as we age in the modern world. What we see is, in fact, abnormal aging, deterioration along the spectrum from fully optimized function and health to disease. It is not a natural consequence of getting chronologically older. Functional medicine is the *medicine of why*. By addressing the imbalances in the body's core biological systems and dynamically interacting networks, you will reverse the hallmarks of aging, feel better quickly, and live a vital, full, long life.

At sixty-three I feel like I am twenty-five years old, except I have more wisdom and meaning and a beautiful community of friends. My body is stronger than ever, and I feel more energetic, challenged, and motivated. I feel as though I am just beginning my journey. My biological age is forty-three. How can you, too, become biologically decades younger than your chronological age?

The key is to address imbalances in your diet and lifestyle—what you have too much or too little of—and in your seven core biological systems through changes that restore balance and health:

- Eat a longevity diet
- Optimize communication and hormonal balance
- Clean up and boost your energy production system
- Cool off inflammation
- Restore the health of your gut and microbiome
- Eliminate or reduce toxic exposures and learn how to optimize detoxification
- Strengthen your muscles, bones, and cells
- Support your circulatory and lymph systems
- Restore balance in your mind, heart, and spirit

The Young Forever Program is founded on sound science translated into simple practices available to almost everyone. Some of the more advanced diagnostics and therapies available may not be covered by insurance or easily available, but they will be soon. Decoding your genome cost $100 billion (£85 billion) in the year 2000. Today, only two decades later, it costs about $1,000 (£850) and soon will be able to be done at home for $100 (£85).

The surprising fact is that if you address the root causes of the hallmarks of aging and disease, then you don't have to treat all the diseases of aging separately. Heart disease, high blood pressure, stroke, dementia, type 2 diabetes, cancer, autoimmune disease, in fact, all disease except acute injury and trauma results from imbalances in the core systems. Get those systems sorted and nearly all diseases go away.

The Young Forever Program is designed to optimize your exposome through a longevity diet full of phytonutrients that mimics calorie restriction, the right type of exercise, deep rest and restoration, good sleep and balanced circadian rhythms, connection, community, and meaning. These are supercharged with the right supplements, and hormetic therapies such as saunas or hot baths, cold showers or cold plunges, red-light therapy, and maybe even hyperbaric oxygen therapy, ozone treatments, and low oxygen simulators if you choose to try them.

You will also learn about emerging treatments for longevity, including NAD+ or its precursors, such as NMN, exosomes, peptides, plasma exchange, natural killer cell infusions, and stem cell therapy. Many of these are out of reach today but will soon become part of the age-reversal tool kit.

HOW TO USE THE YOUNG FOREVER PROGRAM

Building a house starts with a foundation. The same is true for your health. Following are guidelines for how to best use the Young Forever Program, whether you are just starting out or are an advanced longevity bio-adventurer. The key is to build on simple practices that become part of your daily habits and slowly incorporate as much of the advanced testing and supplements as you are able. This road map will best get you to your destination: a long and healthy life.

1. Identify your seven core physiological imbalances through the Young Forever Quizzes (Chapter 13), and, when indicated, get any additional functional medicine testing through a functional medicine practitioner.

2. Get a baseline panel of longevity laboratory testing through your doctor or the Young Forever Function Health Panel (not available in the UK) discussed in Chapter 13.

3. Consider getting a quantified-self biometric device such as an Oura Ring, Garmin, Whoop, Fitbit, Apple Watch, or Levels Health blood sugar monitor, which tracks your blood sugar, blood pressure, heart rate, heart rate variability, sleep, activity, blood oxygen, and more.

4. Explore testing for biological age (DNA methylation, telomeres, immune age testing) as well as advanced screening for cancer and disease through liquid biopsies and full-body MRIs, and for hidden heart disease through AI-driven heart scans.

5. Start the Young Forever Longevity Diet in Chapter 14.

6. Add the Young Forever Supplements for Longevity in Chapter 15.

7. Start making Dr Hyman's Healthy Aging Shake (Chapter 14).

8. Incorporate the Young Forever Lifestyle Practices (exercise, sleep, mind, body, spirit, and hormesis) in Chapter 16.

9. Explore advanced longevity practices and regenerative medicine.

10. Optimize the seven core biological systems by following the personalized advice in Chapter 17. (This may require further testing and treatment with a functional medicine doctor. Go to the Institute for Functional Medicine website, ifm.org, to find one near you.)

You will slowly start to shift your daily habits to include the foundational age-reversing behaviors in the Young Forever Program: the phytochemical-rich longevity diet, the right exercise, sleep optimization, stress-discharging strategies, finding your why and your community. Layer on the longevity supplements, including additional support for any imbalances in your core biological systems and imbalances or deficiencies uncovered through testing. Add simple hormesis practices.

Try advanced longevity-enhancing strategies when you can, such as ozone, hyperbaric oxygen therapy, and peptides. For the adventurous, consider exosomes, plasma exchange, natural killer cell infusions, and stem cell therapy. Use regenerative medicine to fix and heal pain and old injuries. Heal any traumas and your mind, heart, and soul by exploring emerging tools such as dynamic neural retraining, ketamine therapy, stellate ganglion block, and soon-to-be-available treatment with MDMA (also known as Ecstasy) and psilocybin (more to come in Chapter 17 on all these ways of healing the mind, heart, and soul).

Chapter 18 describes my own longevity program—the exact diet, exercise, hormesis practices, supplements, and spiritual routine that I follow to stay healthy and give myself the best chance of living to 120 and beyond and disease-free.

Each person will have a different appetite for exploring these longevity strategies. Some may want to go all in, doing every test and adding in all the therapies. Some may just want to focus on a longevity lifestyle and a few supplements. Do what feels right.

Now, let's get started.

Chapter 13

The Young Forever Program: Testing

Doctors are men who prescribe medicine of which they know little, to cure diseases of which they know less, for human beings of which they know nothing.

—Attributed to Voltaire

We are finally moving into an era of understanding disease, aging, and diagnostic testing that advances beyond Voltaire's cynical admonition about medicine. How can we measure the effect of any approach to promoting health and longevity? How do we know if the changes we make in our lifestyle, supplements, or medications are having a measurable difference on our rate of aging? We have many indirect markers, such as blood sugar, insulin, cholesterol, blood pressure, and other important metrics, that collectively provide a robust picture of the state of our biological networks. When your doctor checks your lab tests, they may check twenty to fifty or even one hundred different analytes. If they are normal, you are given a clean bill of health. However, many of these are surrogate markers. For example, measuring your cholesterol doesn't tell you much about your actual state of health; it is just a predictor of good or bad outcomes based on the numbers. Unfortunately, the vast majority of what's occurring in your body is not even measured or assessed in medical practice.

It reminds me of the old joke about the man who was searching for his keys under a light post. His friend asked him what he was doing. "Looking for my keys," he replied.

"Well, where did you lose them?" the friend asked.

"Down the street."

"Why are you looking here, then?" the friend asked.

"The light is better here," the man replied.

The joke reflects a fundamental problem in medicine. We tend to look at the easily available things but not the most important things.

Functional medicine provides a road map for deep diagnosis and testing of our biological systems—our gut, our immune system, our mitochondria, our detoxification system, our circulatory system, our communications system, and even our structural system. It is excellent at identifying the impediments to health noted previously and deficiencies of the ingredients for health. Through mapping these metrics, we can personalize our self-care and medical care.

The first part of this chapter explains the Young Forever Function Health Panel, which comprises all the recommended lab tests to assess your baseline biological age and health status. Then we review how to assess imbalances in your seven core biological systems using self-assessment quizzes. If you identify imbalances, you may want to explore additional testing. Finally, you may want to consider newer testing for biological and immune system age as well as more sensitive cancer and heart disease screening.

Most of what you need to know can be identified through the Young Forever Longevity Quizzes, but sometimes additional diagnosis and support are needed. You can find a functional medicine practitioner to guide you in the assessment, diagnosis, and treatment of your imbalances at the website for the Institute for Functional Medicine (ifm.org). This chapter also includes recommendations for more advanced testing to further assess imbalances identified by the quizzes when needed. Start by working on the systems with the greatest imbalances, then continue to optimize each out-of-balance biological system over time.

The tools and resources for all the elements of the Young Forever Program would require another book to include and explain. Thank

God for websites. At youngforeverbook.com/resources you will find everything you need to go deeper into the specific tests, supplements, products, and brands that can help you build your own plan.

DIAGNOSING UNDERLYING IMBALANCES AND AGING IN BIOLOGICAL NETWORKS

To start, the following are key basic tests that everyone should get. They will provide you with an overall picture of your health and reveal which of your core systems need better support and additional testing.

Young Forever Function Health Panel

A new company, Function Health (functionhealth.com), gives you access to a complete set of tests at a low cost with periodic retesting every six to twelve months to measure your progress. You don't need a doctor to order these tests. I believe so much in the democratization of health care and helping people learn about their bodies and own their data, which is why I am cofounder (along with Jonathan Swerdlin, Pranitha Patil, Mike Nemke, and Seth Weisfeld) and chief medical officer for the company.

I designed the Young Forever Function Health Panel to create a baseline picture of your health. But the interpretation of these tests is often quite different from how your conventionally trained doctor would interpret them. Most lab reference ranges for "normal" or the "average" in a population are not what is ideal. They are "normal" in the context of a generally unhealthy population. So if you were a Martian landing in America today, you would think it's normal to be overweight. "Normal" fasting blood sugar is 70 to 100 mg/dL. But the fact is that any fasting level over 85 mg/dL increases your risk of heart attack and stroke.

With Function Health, I have created a guide that uses the functional medicine lens to give you insights about your specific test results based on optimal levels and to assess what is wrong and how to fix it. Over time, we will apply artificial intelligence to your long-term results to uncover what doctors may miss. These tests can be ordered by your doctor and may be covered by insurance, but your doctor may not order all of them (because they may not be familiar with them or think they are unnecessary). And they will likely cost a lot more if done through conventional insurance or health care, which may reject paying for the tests and leave you with a bill from the lab at full cost. That is why we built Function Health: to make low-cost testing available to everyone, with a clear interpretative guide we created to empower people with actionable information.

The Young Forever Function Health Panel includes the following tests:

- Complete blood count: red cells, white cells, and platelets
- Urinalysis
- Blood type: ABO
- Kidney function: BUN, creatinine, microalbumin
- Liver function: ALT, AST, GGT, bilirubin, alkaline phosphatase, total protein, albumin
- Pancreatic function: amylase, lipase
- Electrolytes: sodium, potassium, chloride, carbon dioxide
- Sex hormones: for men and women—FSH, LH, testosterone, estradiol, progesterone, prolactin; for women—anti-Mullerian hormone (AMH)
- Prostate health: total and free PSA or prostate-specific antigen
- Adrenal function: cortisol, DHEA-S
- Autoimmunity: antinuclear antibodies, rheumatoid factor
- Inflammation: high-sensitivity C-reactive protein and sedimentation rate
- Metabolic health: glucose, insulin, adiponectin, leptin, hemoglobin A1c, uric acid
- Cardiovascular health: total cholesterol, HDL, LDL, triglycerides, Apo B and A-1, lipoprotein (a) and lipoprotein fractionation for particle number and size, and apolipoprotein E genotype (which assess risk of both cardiovascular disease and dementia)

- Thyroid function: thyroid-stimulating hormone (TSH), free thyroxine (T4), free triiodothyronine (T3), thyroglobulin antibodies (TgAb), thyroid peroxidase antibodies (TPO)
- Toxin exposure: mercury and lead
- Nutritional health: homocysteine, methylmalonic acid (MMA), omega-3 and omega-6 fats, vitamin D, iron studies, zinc, red blood cell magnesium

These tests provide a foundational assessment of your health. They can often cost more than \$15,000 (£12,600), but Function Health provides them for \$499 (£419) as part of a membership. This is the easiest way to get all these tests without waiting for doctor appointments or trying to understand your results in a brief doctor's visit. Function Health also makes it simple to test for cancer through a liquid biopsy with the Galleri test, biological age testing through TruDiagnostic, and your immunological age with Edifice Health's iAge test (more on those later in this chapter). Function Health also provides testing for gluten sensitivity and celiac (including testing for IgA and IgG antigliadin antibodies, IgG and IgA tissue transglutaminase antibodies, and total IgA antibodies), which I think nearly everyone needs.

I recommend everyone get the Young Forever Function Health Panel. Visit functionhealth.com and use the promo code YOUNG FOREVER (membership not currently available in the UK).

Genetic Testing

You have 20,000 genes and 2 to 5 million variations in those genes. That's a lot of data, and much of it scientists are still deciphering. However, there are some genes, or gene variations we call SNPs, or single nucleotide polymorphisms, that are common, clinically meaningful, and modifiable. In these variations, for example, swapping out a T for an A may slightly change the function of that gene. These are modifiable by diet, supplement, and lifestyle changes. Knowing your unique gene variations can help you design a personalized program to lower your risk of disease and increase your chances of a long, healthy life.

A number of companies offer genetic testing. I often use a company called Nordic Laboratories (nordiclabs.com), which provides panels of genes that look at your lipid metabolism, methylation or B vitamin pathways, inflammation, detoxification, oxidative stress, bone health, metabolism, nutrient needs, and screens for celiac genes, iron storage disease, and lactose intolerance. Their panels also look at nutrigenomics, which can help customize your diet, "exercisomics," which can help you optimize exercise, and even genes that determine your risk for mood disorders and mental illness.

DNA Health by Nordic Labs or 3X4 Genetics are the panels I use most often with my patients as the first step in personalizing their health plans. For example, I know I have genes that make it hard for me to detoxify, and to methylate well. Now I add in extra support for detoxification, including supplements, herbs, and regular use of saunas, and I take a stack of B vitamins designed to optimize methylation. This test needs to be ordered and interpreted through your doctor.

QUANTIFIED-SELF METRICS

One of the most exciting developments in medicine is the democratization and decentralization of our health data through the quantified-self movement, the wearable or implantable devices that can measure our real-time functional health. Wearables such as the Oura Ring, Apple Watch, Garmin, Whoop, and Fitbit help you track your heart rate, temperature, heart rate variability, REM sleep, deep sleep, oxygen saturation, EKG, exercise, and need for recovery. Smart beds such as the Eight Sleep provide ways to customize your sleeping temperature, then measure your sleep quality through sensors implanted in the bed.

Implantable devices are also coming fast, starting with the continuous glucose monitor. Considering that 93 percent of Americans are metabolically unhealthy on the spectrum of pre-diabetes to type 2 diabetes, this is something all Americans should do to learn about their bodies. Continuous glucose monitors can measure your unique response to food. Glucose spikes and the resulting insulin surges are important drivers of disease and aging (see "Hallmark 1" in Chapter 4). Using one for a few months or longer can help you identify which foods work and which don't for your body. Levels Health provides an easy-to-use app-enabled glucose monitor to continuously track your blood sugar. As a *Young Forever* reader, you can get access to Levels at levelshealth.com/hyman. A similar system is available from FreeStyle Libre.

Improvements in wearables and implantables will soon allow us to measure more biomarkers in real time, including insulin, inflammation, and potentially thousands of molecules in your body that determine your health. There are even breath analyzers that measure exhaled volatile organic compounds produced by the body that can detect seventeen different diseases, including two types of Parkinson's disease, Crohn's, multiple sclerosis, kidney disease, and cancers like lung, colorectal, prostate, ovarian cancer, and even COVID.[1]

Many converging technologies are about to revolutionize medicine and health care. Soon you will be able to sync your data with your medical history, conventional and functional medicine lab data, and your genome, microbiome, metabolome, proteome, immunome, and transcriptome (all important measures of your gene expression patterns and health). All that data will be organized and interpreted through massive, big-data analytics, maybe even driven by quantum computing informed by machine learning and artificial intelligence filtered through the lens of functional medicine. This will help doctors and individuals make sense of the full complexities of human biology. We can then design real-time personalized strategies and treatments that will radically change how we practice medicine and allow us to implement plans that will help us prevent and reverse disease and dramatically extend health span and life span.

The future is coming fast.

Now, let's get started on the Young Forever Program and translate what you have learned so far into practical steps and daily habits that will help you not only live longer but feel better now, and quickly, so you can meet your life fully present, alive, healthy, and connected to what matters to you.

FUNCTIONAL MEDICINE TESTING: EXPLORING THE SEVEN CORE BIOLOGICAL SYSTEMS

Over the past 30 years, I have been privileged to dive deep into the world of diagnosis through detailed medical histories and extensive functional medicine testing that looks at what conventional medicine often ignores or misses, including nutritional status, microbiome and gut function, food-sensitivity testing, infection testing, mitochondrial assessment, toxic load, detoxification function, deep hormonal analysis, stress hormones, and more.

As a baseline, use the following self-assessments to identify which of your seven core biological systems requires the most focus. Then, in Chapter 17, I will guide you through how to address abnormalities or imbalances uncovered by the quizzes and tests. Most imbalances can be resolved through self-care practices and don't require a doctor. Some, however, may require the help of a good functional medicine doctor to further test for the imbalances in the seven core biological systems.

Scoring the Quizzes

Scoring the quizzes is easy. Just add up the total positive answers and divide by the number of questions, then multiply by 100. That will give the percentage of positive answers. For example, if 12 out of 20 questions are positive, your score is $12 \div 20 = 0.6$. Then multiply 0.6 by 100. Your score is 60 percent.

Core System 1: Testing Your Assimilation, Digestion, and Microbiome

Take the following quiz to assess your inner tube of life. Check each statement that applies to you.

Medical History	Score
I have a bloated or full feeling and/or belching, burning, or flatulence right after meals.	
I have chronic yeast or fungal infections (jock itch, vaginal yeast infection, athlete's foot, toenail fungus).	
I feel nauseated after taking supplements.	
I feel fatigued after eating.	
I have heartburn.	
I regularly use antacids.	
I have chronic abdominal pains.	
I have diarrhea.	
I have constipation (going less than once or twice a day).	
I have greasy, large, poorly formed, or foul-smelling stools.	
I find food that is not fully digested in my stool.	
I have food allergies, intolerance, or reactions.	
I have an intolerance to carbohydrates (eating bread or other sugars causes bloating).	
I have thrush (whitish tongue).	
I have anal itching.	
I have bleeding gums or gingivitis.	
I have geographic tongue (map-like rash on tongue indicating food allergy or yeast overgrowth).	
I have sores on my tongue.	
I have canker sores.	
I crave sweets and bread.	
I drink more than 3 alcoholic beverages a week.	
I have excessive stress.	

I frequently use or have frequently used antibiotics in the past (more than 1–2 times in 3 years).	
I have a history of NSAID (ibuprofen, naproxen, etc.) or other anti-inflammatory use.	
I have taken birth control pills or hormone replacements.	
I have taken prednisone or cortisone.	

I have a family history of any of the following diseases or conditions:
  Autism
  ADHD
  Rosacea
  Acne after adolescence
  Eczema
  Psoriasis
  Celiac disease (gluten allergy)
  Chronic autoimmune diseases
  Chronic hives or urticaria
  Inflammatory bowel disease
  Irritable bowel syndrome
  Chronic fatigue syndrome
  Fibromyalgia	

Your Score

Add the number of positive answers, divide by the number of questions (27), then multiply by 100.

<10 percent. Healthy.

10–50 percent. Moderate imbalances. Follow the guidelines in the Young Forever Program, Chapter 17.

>50 percent. Severe imbalances. Find a functional medicine practitioner to get further testing and support (consult the website of the Institute for Functional Medicine, ifm.org).

Digestive Health Lab Testing

While many labs are offering microbiome analysis, they often look only at the microbes, not the whole picture of what's going on in your gut. The main test I use is called the comprehensive GI Effects test from Genova Diagnostics. The test measures your digestive enzyme function; absorption; gut inflammation and immune function; short-chain fatty acids; microbiome analysis; and stool culture for healthy bacteria, harmful bacteria, yeast, parasites, and worms.

I also use a test from Cyrex Laboratories (Array 2) to measure leaky gut by looking at antibodies to bacterial toxins and zonulin.

Core System 2: Testing Your Immune and Inflammatory System

Take the following quiz to find out if your body is inflamed. Check each statement that applies to you.

Medical History	Score
I have seasonal or environmental allergies.	
I have food allergies or sensitivities, or I don't feel well after eating (sluggishness, headaches, confusion, etc.).	
I work in an environment with poor lighting, chemicals, and/or poor ventilation.	
I am exposed to pesticides, toxic chemicals, loud noise, heavy metals, and/or toxic bosses and coworkers.	
I get frequent colds and infections.	
I have a history of chronic infections such as hepatitis, skin infections, canker sores, and/or cold sores.	
I have sinusitis and allergies.	
I have a family history of bronchitis or asthma.	
I have dermatitis (eczema, acne, rashes).	
I suffer from arthritis (osteoarthritis/degenerative wear and tear).	
I have a family history of autoimmune disease (rheumatoid arthritis, lupus, hypothyroidism, etc.).	
I have a family history of colitis or inflammatory bowel disease.	
I have a family history of irritable bowel syndrome (spastic colon).	

I have depression, anxiety, ADHD, or bipolar disease (brain inflammation).	
I have had a heart attack or have a family history of heart disease.	
I am overweight (BMI greater than 25) or have a family history of obesity or diabetes.	
I have a family history of Parkinson's or Alzheimer's.	
I have a stressful life.	
I drink more than 3 glasses of alcohol a week.	
I exercise less than 30 minutes 3 times a week.	

Your Score

Add the number of positive answers, divide by the number of questions (20), then multiply by 100.

<10 percent. Healthy.

10–50 percent. Moderate imbalances. Follow the guidelines in the Young Forever Program, Chapter 17.

>50 percent. Severe imbalances. Find a functional medicine practitioner to get further testing and support (consult the website of the Institute for Functional Medicine, ifm.org).

Immune/Inflammatory Lab Testing

Many of the markers measured on the Young Forever Function Health Panel (which are also available through most labs and can be ordered by your doctor) assess inflammation, including white blood cell counts, C-reactive protein, sedimentation rate, celiac antibodies, antinuclear antibodies, rheumatoid antibodies, and thyroid antibodies.

For deeper testing of inflammation and the causes of inflammation, functional medicine doctors also look at food sensitivity testing, more advanced autoimmune testing, and infection testing for tick-borne diseases, viruses, and bacteria. We also look at the gut, metabolic health, and toxic load because those can all trigger inflammation.

The most common tests to assess these factors are:

Celiac Antibody Testing

This test measures gluten antibodies including IgA and IgG anti-gliadin antibodies, IgG and IgA tissue transglutaminase antibodies, and total IgA antibodies.

Wheat/Gluten Proteome Reactivity and Autoimmunity: Array 3X from Cyrex Labs

This test measures antibodies to more than twenty wheat and gluten antigens. It is very good at assessing non–celiac gluten sensitivity, which may affect up to 20 percent of the population but is often missed.

Gluten-Associated Cross-Reactive Foods and Foods Sensitivity: Array 4 from Cyrex Labs

If you have gluten sensitivity, then eliminating gluten might not be enough. There are often cross-reactions to other foods, including dairy, eggs, and other grains.

Multiple Food Immune Reactivity Screen: Array 10 from Cyrex Labs

Most food allergy testing looks at the part of immune system that causes true allergy, such as anaphylaxis from peanuts, and measures just IgE antibodies. But you have other antibodies in your immune system defenses. Low-grade delayed food reactions are common, especially for those with a leaky gut. This test measures IgA and IgG antibodies that pick up more subtle reactions to food.

Infection Testing

Doctors generally use antibody testing for infections, but these tests often reflect past infections and do not measure active ones, unless they are PCR tests, like those used to detect COVID-19. Newer tests look at how your white blood cells respond in a culture to the infective agent. We use these tests to determine the level of infection with certain viruses, such as Epstein–Barr or cytomegalovirus, and with tick-borne infections (Lyme, *Ehrlichia*, *Babesia*, *Bartonella*, etc.), which can cause autoimmunity and many other diseases. At my practice, the UltraWellness Center, we often use ArminLabs to assess underlying infections.

Core System 3: Testing Your Energy and Mitochondria

Take the following quiz to see if you may be losing energy. Check each statement that applies to you.

Medical History	Score
I have chronic or prolonged fatigue.	
I have muscle pain or discomfort.	
I have sleep problems (trouble staying or falling asleep or waking up early).	
My sleep is not refreshing.	
I have a poor tolerance to exercise, with severe fatigue after.	
I have muscle weakness.	
I have trouble concentrating or with memory.	
I am irritable and moody.	
Fatigue prevents me from doing things I would like to do.	
Fatigue interferes with work, family, or social life.	
I have been under prolonged stress.	
My symptoms started after an acute stress incident, infection, or trauma.	
I have chronic fatigue syndrome or fibromyalgia.	
I have a history of chronic infections.	
I overeat.	
I have been exposed to environmental chemicals (pesticides, unfiltered water, nonorganic food).	

Medical History	Score
I served in the Gulf War or another military engagement and have suffered negative consequences.	
I have a family history of neurological diseases, including Alzheimer's, Parkinson's, ALS, etc.	
I have a family history of autism or ADHD.	
I have a family history of depression, bipolar disease, or schizophrenia.	

Your Score

Add the number of positive answers, divide by the number of questions (20), then multiply by 100.

<10 percent. Healthy.

10–50 percent. Moderate imbalances. Follow the guidelines in the Young Forever Program, Chapter 17.

>50 percent. Severe imbalances. Find a functional medicine practitioner to get further testing and support (consult the website of the Institute for Functional Medicine, ifm.org).

Mitochondria Lab Testing

Conventional medicine pretty much draws a blank in assessing your mitochondria and energy system. Some tests such as muscle biopsies or functional MRI scans can assess mitochondrial function and health but are only used by specialists looking for rare disorders.

However, there are a few simple ways to assess mitochondrial health:

Oxidative Stress Testing

Conventional labs can look at markers of oxidative stress, including F2-isoprostanes, myeloperoxidase, and oxidized LDL.

Genova's Oxidative Stress Analysis 2.0 is a more comprehensive assessment that measures urine 8-hydroxy-deoxy guanosine, which reveals any damage to your DNA. Blood markers include glutathione total antioxidant capacity, glutathione peroxidase, superoxide dismutase, and lipid peroxides (oxidized fat).

The NutrEval nutritional panel from Genova Diagnostics also measures antioxidant levels, including coenzyme 10, vitamins E and A, and beta-carotene.

The DNA Health test by Nordic Labs measures a panel of antioxidant genes that can identify poor antioxidant capacity.

Organic Acid Testing

The best test for mitochondrial function is the organic acid test. I use the Organix profile by Genova Diagnostics. It measures the Krebs cycle metabolites, identifying any dysfunction in the process of turning food and oxygen into ATP, the body's energy source.

VO_2 Max Testing

The other metric commonly used to assess mitochondrial function measures the rate at which you can burn oxygen and calories. It is called the VO_2 max test and is highly correlated with fitness and longevity. It is performed by many gyms or in hospitals that have a metabolic unit. Wearing a mask that measures oxygen consumed and carbon dioxide expelled, you run or bike as fast as you can for as long as you can. The VO_2 max is measured in liters of oxygen consumed per minute. The more liters you can burn per minute, the more calories you burn per minute, the faster your metabolism, and the healthier your mitochondria. Diabetics have very low rates, often under 20, and elite athletes have VO_2 max rates over 80.

Core System 4: Testing Your Detoxification System

Take the following quiz to find out if you are at risk for toxin overload. Check each statement that applies to you.

Medical History	Score
I have hard, difficult-to-pass bowel movements every day or every other day.	
I am constipated and only go every other day or less often.	
I urinate small amounts of dark, strong-smelling urine only a few times a day.	
I almost never break a real sweat.	
I experience one or more of the following: 　Fatigue 　Muscle aches 　Headaches 　Concentration and memory problems	
I have a family history of fibromyalgia or chronic fatigue syndrome.	
I drink unfiltered tap or well water or water from plastic bottles.	
I dry-clean my clothes.	
I work or live in a building with poor ventilation or windows that don't open.	
I live in a large urban or industrial area.	
I use household or lawn and garden chemicals or get my house or apartment treated for bugs by an exterminator.	
I have more than 1–2 mercury amalgams (fillings) in my teeth.	
I eat large fish (swordfish, tuna, shark, tilefish) more than once a week.	
I am bothered by one or more of the following: 　Petrol or diesel fumes 　Perfumes 　New car smell 　Fabric stores 　Dry-cleaned clothes 　Hair spray 　Other strong odors 　Soaps 　Detergents 　Tobacco smoke 　Chlorinated water	

I have a negative reaction when I consume foods containing MSG, sulfites (found in wine, salad bars, dried fruit), sodium benzoate (preservative), red wine, cheese, bananas, chocolate, garlic, onions, or even a small amount of alcohol.	
When I drink caffeine, I feel wired, experience an increase in joint and muscle aches, and/or have hypoglycemic symptoms (anxiety, palpitations, sweating, dizziness).	
I regularly consume any of the following substances or medications: Acid-blocking drugs Hormone-modulating medications in pills, patches, or creams (the birth control pill, estrogen, progesterone, prostate medication) Ibuprofen or naproxen Medications for recurrent headaches, allergy symptoms, nausea, diarrhea, or indigestion Paracetamol	
I have had jaundice (skin and whites of eyes turning yellow) or I have been told I have Gilbert's syndrome (an elevation of bilirubin).	
I have a family history of any of the following conditions: Breast cancer Smoking-induced lung cancer Other type of cancer Prostate problems Food allergies, sensitivities, or intolerances	
I have a family history of Parkinson's, Alzheimer's, ALS (amyotrophic lateral sclerosis), or other motor neuron diseases, or multiple sclerosis.	

Your Score

Add up the number of positive answers, divide by the number of questions (20), then multiply by 100.

<10 percent. Healthy.

10–50 percent. Moderate imbalances. Follow the guidelines in the Young Forever Program, Chapter 17.

>50 percent. Severe imbalances. Find a functional medicine practitioner to get further testing and support (consult the website of the Institute for Functional Medicine, ifm.org).

Detoxification Lab Testing

The Young Forever Function Health Panel includes kidney and liver tests that look for more severe dysfunction. By the time your kidney tests are abnormal, you have lost 50 percent of your kidney function. When your liver tests are abnormal, your liver cells are already dying. While our conventional labs are good at picking up serious problems, they miss early-stage imbalances in your detoxification system.

It is worth mentioning that one of the liver tests, gamma-glutamyl transpeptidase (GGT), can identify environmental toxin exposure and fatty liver. GGT can be elevated in people with insulin resistance, pre-diabetes or type 2 diabetes, drug exposures, excess alcohol intake, and exposure to environmental toxins.

Urine protein levels measured by microalbumin (also part of the Young Forever Function Health Panel) can be helpful in picking up early kidney damage from high blood pressure, diabetes, or other kidney diseases.

The organic acid tests and oxidative stress analysis mentioned on pages 186–7 are also helpful in assessing your detoxification ability, especially the status of glutathione, the body's main detoxifying molecule. The DNA Health test and the 3X4 Genetics test measure a profile of detoxifying genes, which can identify poor detox capacity.

Heavy Metal Testing

Low-level heavy metal toxicity is one of the most common and undiagnosed causes of a whole host of diseases, including heart disease, cancer, diabetes, dementia, autoimmune disease, depression, insomnia, fatigue, and more. We all know about lead toxicity in children from eating paint chips or from the Flint, Michigan, water crisis.

Thankfully leaded paint and leaded petrol have been banned. But lead is still ubiquitous and mostly ignored. Blood lead levels over 2 mcg/dL are associated with a higher risk of heart attack and death than abnormal cholesterol. Nearly 40 percent of the population has levels over 2.[2]

Conventional doctors might look at blood levels and might test a 24-hour sample for occupational or acute exposures, but they don't look at metals stored over your lifetime in your muscles, organs, and brain. The Young Forever Function Health Panel measures blood levels, but how do we test for your long-term body burden?

Functional medicine doctors use a chelation challenge test. Genova Diagnostics and Doctor's Data offer excellent versions of this test, looking at the overall burden of toxic heavy metal exposures through the urine toxic element test. An FDA-approved chemical chelation agent called DMSA can be used to mobilize the metals that are found in a 6-hour urine sample. This is called a heavy metal challenge test. The usual dose is 3 mg/kg of DMSA or about 1,500 mg for the challenge dose.

Quicksilver Scientific offers a unique blood, hair, and urine test called the Mercury Tri-Test, which measures both organic mercury (primarily from fish consumption) and inorganic mercury (from dental fillings and pollution). It also measures the effectiveness of mercury detoxification via hair and urine.

Mold Toxicity

Another mostly ignored load of toxins comes from mold and the mycotoxins they produce.

Thirty to fifty percent of buildings in the United States have water damage and contain some level of mold. There are 200 types of mold that present serious health risks to humans or animals. These harmful species are known as toxic molds and produce potentially dangerous mycotoxins that can cause many medical conditions and symptoms. MyMycoLab tests for IgE and IgG antibodies to mold toxins and can screen for mold exposure.

Fatty Liver Scan

About 25 percent of the American population has a fatty liver. That is more than 80 million people, and almost all have no idea.[3] You might have it even if your liver function test results are "normal." Fatty liver drives heart disease, cancer, type 2 diabetes, dementia, and more. It is caused by sugar and starch in our diet. The best test is a liver MRI (which is included in the total-body MRI scans now available; see page 217). A liver ultrasound or FibroScan can also help identify a fatty liver.

Core System 5: Testing Your Communication and Hormone Balance

Insulin Resistance

Take the following quiz to find out if you have less-than-optimal insulin or blood sugar levels. Check each statement that applies to you.

Medical History	Score
I crave sweets and eat them, and though I get a temporary boost of energy and mood, I later crash.	
I have a family history of diabetes, hypoglycemia, or alcoholism.	
I get irritable, anxious, tired, and jittery, or get headaches intermittently throughout the day, but feel better temporarily after meals.	
I feel shaky 2–3 hours after a meal.	
I eat a low-fat diet but can't seem to lose weight.	
If I miss a meal, I feel cranky and irritable, weak, or tired.	
If I eat a carbohydrate breakfast (muffin, bagel, cereal, pancakes, etc.), I can't seem to control my eating for the rest of the day.	
Once I start eating sweets or carbohydrates, I can't seem to stop.	
If I eat fish or meat and vegetables, I feel good, but I seem to get sleepy or feel "drugged" after eating a meal full of pasta, bread, potatoes, and dessert.	

I go for the bread basket at restaurants.	
I get heart palpitations after eating sweets.	
I seem salt-sensitive (I tend to retain water).	
I get panic attacks in the afternoon if I skip breakfast.	
I am often moody, impatient, or anxious.	
My memory and concentration are poor.	
Eating makes me calm.	
I get tired a few hours after eating.	
I get night sweats.	
I am tired most of the time.	
I have extra weight around my middle (waist-to-hip ratio >0.8; measure around the belly button and around the bony prominence at the front of the top of the hip).	
My hair thins in the places I don't want it to (my head) and it grows in the places it shouldn't (my face, if I am a woman).	
I have a family history of polycystic ovarian syndrome or am infertile.	
I have a family history of high blood pressure.	
I have a family history of heart disease.	
I have a family history of type 2 diabetes.	
I have chronic fungal infections (jock itch, vaginal yeast infections, dry, scaly patches on my skin).	

Your Score

Add up the number of positive answers, divide by the number of questions (26), then multiply by 100.

<10 percent. Healthy.

10–50 percent. Moderate imbalances. Follow the guidelines in the Young Forever Program, Chapter 17.

>50 percent. Severe imbalances. Find a functional medicine practitioner to get further testing and support (consult the website of the Institute for Functional Medicine, ifm.org).

Sex Hormone Imbalances for Women

Take the following quiz to find out if your sex hormones are out of balance. Check each statement that applies to you.

Medical History	Score
I have premenstrual syndrome.	
I have monthly weight fluctuation.	
I have edema, swelling, puffiness, or water retention.	
I feel bloated.	
I have headaches.	
I have mood swings.	
I have tender, enlarged breasts.	
I have a poor mood.	
I feel unable to cope with ordinary demands.	
I have backaches, joint, or muscle pain.	
I have premenstrual food cravings (especially sugar or salt).	
I have irregular cycles, heavy bleeding, or light bleeding.	
I am infertile.	
I use birth control pills or other hormones.	
I have premenstrual migraines.	
I have breast cysts or lumps or fibrocystic breasts.	
I have a family history of breast, ovarian, or uterine cancer.	
I have a family history of uterine fibroids.	

I have peri- or menopausal symptoms.	
I have hot flushes.	
I feel anxious.	
I have night sweats.	
I have insomnia.	
I have lost my sex drive.	
I have dry skin, hair, and/or vagina.	
I have heart palpitations.	
I have trouble with memory or concentration.	
I have bloating or weight gain around the middle.	
I have facial hair.	
I have been exposed to pesticides or heavy metals (in food, water, air).	

Your Score

Add up the number of positive answers, divide by the number of questions (30), then multiply by 100.

<10 percent. Healthy.

10–50 percent. Moderate imbalances. Follow the guidelines in the Young Forever Program, Chapter 17.

>50 percent. Severe imbalances. Find a functional medicine practitioner to get further testing and support (consult the website of the Institute for Functional Medicine, ifm.org).

Sex Hormone Imbalances for Men

Take the following quiz to find out if your sex hormones are out of balance. Check each statement that applies to you.

Medical History	Score
I have a reduced sex drive and have lost my vitality.	
I have trouble achieving or maintaining an erection.	
I am infertile or have a low sperm count.	
I have loss of muscle.	
I have increased abdominal fat.	
I am fatigued or have low energy.	
I feel a loss of direction and purpose or a sense of apathy.	
I have bone loss or bone fractures.	
I have a family history of high cholesterol.	
I have a family history of insulin or blood sugar problems.	
I feel weak.	
I have a poor mood.	
I have been exposed to pesticides or heavy metals (in food, water, air).	

Your Score

Add up the number of positive answers, divide by the number of questions (13), then multiply by 100.

   <10 percent. Healthy.
   10–50 percent. Moderate imbalances. Follow the guidelines in the Young Forever Program, Chapter 17.
   >50 percent. Severe imbalances. Find a functional medicine practitioner to get help (consult the website of the Institute for Functional Medicine, ifm.org).

Thyroid Imbalance

Take the following quiz to find out if your thyroid is functioning optimally. Check each statement that applies to you.

Medical History	Score
I have thick skin and fingernails.	
I have dry skin.	
My hair is thinning, I lose hair, or I have coarse hair.	
I am sensitive to cold.	
I have cold hands and feet.	
I have muscle fatigue, pain, or weakness.	
I have heavy menstrual bleeding, worsening of premenstrual syndrome, other menstrual problems, or infertility.	
My sex drive has decreased.	
I retain fluid (swelling of hands and feet).	
I feel fatigued (especially in the morning).	
I have low blood pressure and heart rate.	
I have trouble with memory and concentration.	
The outer third of my eyebrows is thinning.	
I have trouble losing weight or have recent weight gain.	
I have constipation.	
I have a poor mood and am apathetic.	
I have a family history of autoimmune disease (such as rheumatoid arthritis, multiple sclerosis, lupus, allergies, yeast overgrowth).	
I have a family history of celiac disease or am gluten-sensitive.	
I have been exposed to radiation treatments.	
I have been exposed to environmental toxins.	
I consume a lot of tuna and sushi and/or have multiple dental silver (mercury) fillings.	
I have a family history of thyroid problems.	
I drink chlorinated or fluoridated water.	

Your Score

Add up the number of positive answers, divide by the number of questions (23), then multiply by 100.

<10 percent. Healthy.

10–50 percent. Moderate imbalances. Follow the guidelines in the Young Forever Program, Chapter 17.

>50 percent. Severe imbalances. Find a functional medicine practitioner to get help (consult the website of the Institute for Functional Medicine, ifm.org).

Communication Health Lab Testing

The Young Forever Function Health Panel covers most of the hormone analysis, including insulin (and blood sugar and hemoglobin A1c), thyroid function, stress hormones (DHEA-S and cortisol), and sex hormones (estrogen, progesterone, testosterone). It also measures your full lipid panel, including a more advanced version than your regular cholesterol tests. It is far more accurate in identifying insulin resistance and the risk of heart attacks by measuring lipid particle number and size.

Additional functional medicine testing may help further identify hormonal imbalances:

The Adrenocortex Stress Profile by Genova Diagnostics measures saliva levels of cortisol, the stress hormone, throughout the day. It can identify high levels of cortisol, which indicate high levels of stress, disruptions in your circadian rhythms, and low levels of cortisol, which indicate adrenal fatigue and burnout. It is best to test cortisol at multiple points throughout the day to ensure that your levels are normal *and* that you have a normal pattern of cortisol release (highest upon waking and lowest before bed). Lifestyle interventions and various supplements can help restore adrenal balance (see Chapter 17).

Essential Estrogens by Genova Diagnostics is a 24-hour urine test that measures estrogens and estrogen metabolites, which are helpful in identifying carcinogenic and dangerous estrogen compounds. These can form from poor diet, genetic predisposition, nutritional deficiencies, and environmental toxins. Lifestyle, herbs, and nutritional supplements can improve estrogen metabolism.

Core System 6: Testing Your Circulatory Health

Take the following quiz to find out if your circulation and lymphatic systems are working efficiently. Check each statement that applies to you.

Medical History	Score
I have heart disease (angina or heart attacks).	
I have high blood pressure.	
I have poor circulation in my feet.	
I get swelling in my hands and feet.	
I have edema.	
I have erectile dysfunction.	
I have muscle cramps.	
I get cold hands and feet.	
I have Raynaud's syndrome.	
I get frequent infections.	
I have varicose veins.	
I get numbness and tingling in my extremities.	
My wounds heal slowly.	
I have blood clots.	

Your Score

Add up the number of positive answers, divide by the number of questions (14), then multiply by 100.

<10 percent. Healthy.

10–50 percent. Moderate imbalances. Follow the guidelines in the
Young Forever Program, Chapter 17.

>50 percent. Severe imbalances. Find a functional medicine prac-
titioner to get further testing and support (consult the website of
the Institute for Functional Medicine, ifm.org).

Circulatory Health Lab Testing

Assessing blood vessel health is important and increasingly easy to do.
Blood pressure is a great indicator of your vascular health and can be
taken at home.

Cleerly, an innovative new heart scan (see page 218), uses artificial
intelligence to measure soft, vulnerable plaque in your arteries using a
high-speed CT scan.

A carotid ultrasound of the arteries in your neck can look for thickening of your blood vessel walls and plaques that could cause a stroke.
It is called a carotid intima-media thickness test.

A full-body MRI (see page 217) can be used to assess the health of
your heart's and brain's blood vessels and check for aneurysms.

Heart rate variability, easily tested with a smart watch, a smart-
phone's camera, or devices like an Oura Ring, measures the health of
your autonomic nervous system, which directly affects your vascular
health. Tests for inflammation and oxidative stress indirectly indicate
potential harm to your blood vessels.

Core System 7: Testing Your Musculoskeletal and Structural System

Take the following quiz to find out if your structural house is healthy.
Check each statement that applies to you.

Medical History	Score
I have lost muscle mass over the years.	
I find it harder to do daily tasks that require strength.	

I don't do strength training.	
I am a vegan.	
I eat less than 25–30 grams of protein per meal.	
I don't eat fish or take omega-3 fatty acid supplements.	
I eat fried foods.	
I have osteopenia or osteoporosis.	
I don't take a vitamin D$_3$ supplement.	
I have low energy and stamina.	

Your Score

Add up the number of positive answers, divide by the number of questions (10), then multiply by 100.

<10 percent. Healthy.

10–50 percent. Moderate imbalances. Follow the guidelines in the Young Forever Program, Chapter 17.

>50 percent. Severe imbalances. Find a functional medicine practitioner to get further testing and support (consult the website of the Institute for Functional Medicine, ifm.org).

Musculoskeletal Health Lab Testing

Examining your musculoskeletal system is complex. But the new total-body MRI scans can provide a good assessment of your general structural health.

The omega index test (part of the Young Forever Function Health Panel) also looks at your fatty acid status. Omega-3 fats are essential building blocks of every cell membrane and your brain. Low levels cause disease.

However, the most important test to assess your overall structural and metabolic health is the DEXA scan, a low-intensity X-ray scan used to measure *bone density* for osteoporosis, an important screening test because osteoporosis can be reversed. But the test also measures your *body composition,* and not only the amount of muscle and fat but where it is located. Many other measures of body composition look at the whole body. But if you have skinny arms and legs and a big belly, you could average out to normal but still be at high risk of aging rapidly and disease. The DEXA scan looks at one of the most important predictors of disease and death: visceral, organ, or belly fat.

An easy home test is the waist-to-hip ratio. Simply measure the widest point around your hips and the widest point around your belly, usually around your belly button. Divide the waist measurement by the hip measurement. If the waist-to-hip ratio is greater than 0.8 for a woman or greater than 0.9 for a man, you likely have high levels of dangerous organ or visceral fat.

TESTING YOUR NUTRITIONAL STATUS

More than 90 percent of us are deficient in one or more nutrients, according to large government studies. The most common deficiencies are omega-3 fats, vitamin D, B vitamins, magnesium, and zinc. Tests for these are part of the Young Forever Function Health Panel, but you can also use these short quizzes to highlight your risk for deficiency.

Essential Fatty Acid Deficiency (Omega-3s)

Take the following quiz to find out if your fatty acids are balanced. Check each statement that applies to you.

Medical History	Score
I have soft, cracked, or brittle nails.	
I have dry, itchy, scaling, or flaking skin.	
I have hard earwax.	
I have chicken skin (tiny bumps on the backs of arms or on the trunk).	

I have dandruff.	
I feel aching or stiffness in my joints.	
I am thirsty most of the time.	
I am constipated (have fewer than 2 bowel movements a day).	
I have light-colored, hard, or foul-smelling stools.	
I have poor mood, difficulty paying attention, and/or memory loss.	
I have high blood pressure.	
I have fibrocystic breasts.	
I have premenstrual syndrome.	
I have a family history of high LDL cholesterol, low HDL levels, and high triglycerides.	
I am of North Atlantic genetic background: Irish, Scottish, Welsh, Scandinavian, or coastal Native American.	

Your Score

Add up the number of positive answers, divide by the number of questions (15), then multiply by 100.

<10 percent. Healthy.
10–50 percent. Moderate imbalances. Follow the guidelines in the Young Forever Program, Chapter 17.
>50 percent. Severe imbalances. Find a functional medicine practitioner to get further testing and support (consult the website of the Institute for Functional Medicine, ifm.org).

Vitamin D Deficiency

Take the following quiz to find out if your vitamin D levels are adequate. Check each statement that applies to you.

Medical History	Score
I have a family history of seasonal affective disorder (SAD) or the winter blues.	
I have experienced a loss of mental sharpness or memory.	
I have sore or weak muscles.	
I have tender bones (press on your shin bone to see if it hurts).	
I work indoors.	
I avoid the sun.	
I wear sunblock most of the time.	
I live north of Florida.	
I don't eat small, fatty fish such as mackerel, herring, or sardines (the main source of dietary vitamin D).	
I have a family history of osteoporosis.	
I have broken more than 2 bones or had a hip fracture.	
I have a family history of autoimmune disease (such as multiple sclerosis).	
I have osteoarthritis.	
I have frequent infections.	
I have a family history of prostate cancer.	
I have dark skin (any race other than Caucasian).	
I am 60 years old or older.	

Your Score

Add up the number of positive answers, divide by the number of questions (17), then multiply by 100.

<10 percent. Healthy.
10–50 percent. Moderate imbalances. Follow the guidelines in the Young Forever Program, Chapter 17.

>50 percent. Severe imbalances. Find a functional medicine practitioner to get further testing and support (consult the website of the Institute for Functional Medicine, ifm.org).

Magnesium Deficiency

Take the following quiz to find out if your magnesium levels are adequate. Check each statement that applies to you.

Medical History	Score
I have a poor mood.	
I feel irritable.	
I have difficulty focusing.	
I have a family history of autism.	
I am anxious.	
I have trouble falling and/or staying asleep.	
I have muscle twitching.	
I have premenstrual syndrome.	
I have leg or hand cramps.	
I have restless leg syndrome.	
I have heart flutters, skipped beats, or palpitations.	
I get frequent headaches or migraines.	
I have trouble swallowing.	
I have acid reflux.	
I am sensitive to loud noises.	
I feel fatigued.	
I have a family history of asthma.	
I have constipation (fewer than 2 bowel movements a day).	
I have excess stress.	
I have kidney stones.	

Medical History	Score
I have a family history of heart disease or heart failure.	
I have a family history of mitral valve prolapse.	
I have a family history of diabetes.	
I have a low intake of kelp, wheat bran or germ, almonds, cashews, buckwheat, or dark-green leafy vegetables.	

Your Score

Add up the number of positive answers, divide by the number of questions (24), then multiply by 100.

<10 percent. Healthy.

10–50 percent. Moderate imbalances. Follow the guidelines in the Young Forever Program, Chapter 17.

>50 percent. Severe imbalances. Find a functional medicine practitioner to get further testing and support (consult the website of the Institute for Functional Medicine, ifm.org).

Zinc Deficiency

Take the following quiz to find out if your zinc levels are inadequate. Check each statement that applies to you.

Medical History	Score
I have impaired taste.	
I have impaired smell.	
I have weak nails (thin, brittle, peeling).	
I have white spots on my nails.	
I have frequent colds or respiratory infections.	
I have diarrhea.	

I have eczema or other skin rashes.	
I have acne.	
My wounds heal poorly.	
I have allergies.	
I am losing my hair.	
I have dandruff.	
I have a family history of erectile dysfunction.	
I have an enlarged or inflamed prostate.	
I have a family history of inflammatory bowel disease (ulcerative colitis, Crohn's disease).	
I have a family history of rheumatoid arthritis.	
I consume hard water (which depletes zinc).	
I consume more than 3 alcoholic beverages per week.	
I sweat excessively.	
I have a family history of kidney or liver disease.	
I am over age 65.	
I use diuretics (water pills).	
I have a low intake of dulse (seaweed), fresh ginger root, egg yolks, fish, kelp, lamb, legumes, and pumpkin seeds.	

Your Score

Add up the number of positive answers, divide by the number of questions (23), then multiply by 100.

<10 percent. Healthy.

10–50 percent. Moderate imbalances. Follow the guidelines in the Young Forever Program, Chapter 17.

>50 percent. Severe imbalances. Find a functional medicine practitioner to get further testing and support (consult the website of the Institute for Functional Medicine, ifm.org).

Methylation Imbalances: B Vitamin Status (B$_{12}$, folate, B$_6$)

Take the following quiz to find out if your methylation function (which depends on vitamins B$_6$, B$_{12}$, and folate) is adequate. Check each statement that applies to you.

Medical History	Score
I eat animal protein (meat of any kind, dairy, cheese, eggs) more than 5 times a week.	
I eat more than 1–2 foods a week with hydrogenated fats (margarine, shortening, processed or packaged foods).	
I have servings of animal protein greater than 115–175 grams (the size of the palm of your hand) at a meal.	
I eat less than 100 grams of dark-green leafy vegetables a day.	
I eat fewer than 5–9 servings (1 serving = 40 grams) of fruits and vegetables a day.	
I have more than 3 alcoholic drinks a week.	
I have a poor mood.	
I have a history of a heart attack or other heart disease.	
I have a history of stroke.	
I have a history of cancer (especially colon, cervix, breast).	
I have a history of abnormal PAP test (cervical dysplasia).	
I have a history of birth defects in offspring (neural tube defects or Down syndrome).	
I have a history of dementia.	
I have a loss of balance or sensation in feet.	
I have a history of multiple sclerosis or other diseases with nerve damage.	
I have a history of carpal tunnel syndrome.	
I do not take a multivitamin.	
I am over 65 years old.	

Your Score

Add up the number of positive answers, divide by the number of questions (18), then multiply by 100.

<10 percent. Healthy.

10–50 percent. Moderate imbalances. Follow the guidelines in the Young Forever Program, Chapter 17.

>50 percent. Severe imbalances. Find a functional medicine practitioner to get further testing and support (consult the website of the Institute for Functional Medicine, ifm.org).

Nutritional Health Lab Testing

Many nutrient levels can be easily measured through conventional tests (on the Young Forever Function Health Panel), including the most common deficiencies in America, such as omega-3 fats, vitamin D, zinc, and iron.

The NutrEval Panel from Genova Diagnostics measures amino acids, fatty acids, vitamins and minerals, antioxidants, and organic acids for a full picture of your nutritional status. This test must be ordered by your functional medicine practitioner.

Stress and Mental Health Assessment

The best screening tests to assess your mental state and health risks from stress are the ACE (Adverse Childhood Experiences) Questionnaire and the Perceived Stress Scale (PSS). It is worth taking a minute to score these tests. Both past adverse experiences and perceived stress levels are highly predictive of your risk of disease and death. Why? The most powerful pharmacy to create health or harm is located between your ears.

The micro- and macrotraumas we all experience directly from our life events and the low-level stress and trauma of living in a world full of conflict, division, racism, sexism, poverty, social isolation, and massive health and economic disparities are an invisible threat to our health. While we can't end war or racism or poverty overnight, we can shift our own relationship to stress and heal our past and present trauma with important new tools (see Chapters 16 and 17). Since our mindset and sense of love and safety are critical determinants of our health and impact everything from our level of happiness and connection to our actual biology—changing our DNA methylation, telomeres, inflammation, microbiome, hormones, muscle mass, energy production, in fact, every function of our body—it is essential for us to heal this part of us.

Take a minute to complete the Perceived Stress Scale and the ACE Quiz.

Perceived Stress Scale

For each question, choose from the following alternatives:[4]
0 = never 1 = almost never 2 = sometimes 3 = fairly often 4 = very often

1. In the last month, how often have you been upset because of something that happened unexpectedly?
2. In the last month, how often have you felt that you were unable to control the important things in your life?
3. In the last month, how often have you felt nervous and stressed?
4. In the last month, how often have you felt confident about your ability to handle your personal problems?
5. In the last month, how often have you felt that things were going your way?
6. In the last month, how often have you found that you could not cope with all the things that you had to do?
7. In the last month, how often have you been able to control irritations in your life?
8. In the last month, how often have you felt that you were on top of things?
9. In the last month, how often have you been angered because of things that happened that were outside of your control?

10. In the last month, how often have you felt difficulties were piling up so high that you could not overcome them?

Figuring Your PSS Score

You can determine your PSS score by following these directions:

- First, reverse your scores for questions 4, 5, 7, and 8. On these 4 questions, change the scores like this: 0 = 4, 1 = 3, 2 = 2, 3 = 1, 4 = 0.
- Now add up your scores for each item to get a total. *My total score is*_____.

Individual scores on the PSS can range from 0 to 40, with higher scores indicating higher perceived stress.
Scores ranging from 0 to 13 would be considered low stress.
Scores ranging from 14 to 26 would be considered moderate stress.
Scores ranging from 27 to 40 would be considered high perceived stress.

The Perceived Stress Scale is important because your *perception* of what is happening in your life is most essential to how your body responds to different stressors. Two individuals could have the exact same events and experiences in their lives, but, depending on their perceptions, the total score could put one of those individuals in the low-stress category and the other in the high-stress category.

Adverse Childhood Experiences (ACE) Questionnaire

For each "yes" answer, add 1. The total is your cumulative number of ACEs.

Before your eighteenth birthday:

1. Did a parent or other adult in the household often or very often: swear at you, insult you, put you down, or humiliate you or act in a way that made you afraid that you might be physically hurt?

2. Did a parent or other adult in the household often or very often: push, grab, slap, or throw something at you or ever hit you so hard that you had marks or were injured?

3. Did an adult or person at least 5 years older than you ever: touch or fondle you or have you touch their body in a sexual way or attempt or have oral, anal, or vaginal intercourse with you?

4. Did you often or very often feel that no one in your family loved you or thought you were important or special? Or that your family didn't look out for each other, feel close to each other, or support each other?

5. Did you often or very often feel that you didn't have enough to eat, had to wear dirty clothes, and had no one to protect you? Or that your parents were too drunk or high to take care of you or take you to the doctor if you needed it?

6. Were your parents ever separated or divorced?

7. Was your mother or stepmother: often or very often pushed, grabbed, slapped, or had something thrown at her; or sometimes, often, or very often kicked, bitten, hit with a fist, or hit with something hard; or ever repeatedly hit over at least a few minutes or threatened with a gun or knife?

8. Did you live with anyone who was a problem drinker or alcoholic, or who used street drugs?

9. Was a household member depressed or mentally ill, or did a household member attempt suicide?

10. Did a household member go to prison?

The ACE Questionnaire is a variation on the questions asked in the original ACE study conducted by CDC researchers.

Two-thirds of the original study participants had a score of at least 1, and of those, 87 percent had a score of 2 or more. As your ACE score increases, so does the risk of disease and social and emotional problems. With an ACE score of 4 or more, things start getting serious. For example, the risk of depression goes up 460 percent and that of suicide 1,220 percent. The life expectancy of an individual with an ACE score of 6 or more may be reduced by up to 20 years. We are all at risk for some level of trauma. Even not being loved and accepted fully as a child (or even as an adult) is a form of microtrauma.

What was not assessed in the ACE study (and are also important stressors)?

- Stressors outside the household (e.g., violence, poverty, racism, other forms of discrimination, isolation, chaotic environment, lack of services)
- Protective factors (e.g., supportive relationships, community services, skill-building opportunities)
- Individual differences (i.e., not all children who experience multiple ACEs will have poor outcomes and not all children who have experienced no ACEs will avoid poor outcomes—a high ACE score is simply an indicator of greater risk)

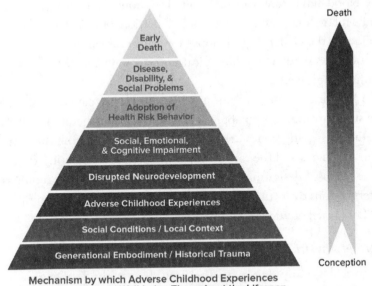

Mechanism by which Adverse Childhood Experiences Influence Health and Well-being Throughout the Lifespan

Source: Centers for Disease Control and Prevention. "About the CDC-Kaiser ACE Study." Last reviewed April 6, 2021. cdc.gov/violenceprevention/aces/about.html.

These factors can create additional trauma that becomes embedded in your biology. Understanding these scores, your levels of stress, and adverse childhood experiences is not a reason for despair but something to address and heal. In Chapters 16 and 17, you will learn powerful new strategies to reset your perceived stress levels and truly heal from trauma.

MEASURING BIOLOGICAL AGING, DISEASE SCREENING, AND ADVANCED DIAGNOSTICS

Much aging research has been hampered because of the lack of good metrics, or tests to track actual biological age. Thankfully this is changing. As we learned in Chapter 3 on biological aging, tests are now available to track our rate of aging. While these tests are not widely available and are unlikely to be ordered by your conventional doctor, home testing kits and kits you can bring to a lab that will do the blood/fluid draw can be ordered without a doctor's prescription and sent to diagnostic companies. Function Health has such tests, including the Galleri liquid biopsy for cancer screening, the TruDiagnostic DNA methylation biological age test, and iAge, the test for your immunological age.

I have used these tests on myself and with my patients. While we are still learning how to apply them in clinical medicine, I find them useful in assessing your current biological age, measuring the status of your telomeres and the rate of inflammaging, and screening for early-stage disease, designing a disease-reversal strategy, and monitoring interventions over time.

Let's briefly review each one.

DNA Methylation: A Measurement of Biological Age

I have done my DNA methylation test with TruDiagnostic, a direct-to-consumer, commercially available test. When I did the test I was sixty-two years old chronologically but only forty-three biologically! Function Health also offers this DNA methylation test.

YOUR EXTRINSIC
Epigenetic Age

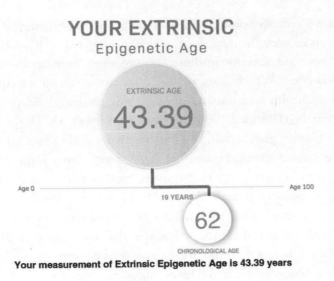

Your measurement of Extrinsic Epigenetic Age is 43.39 years

Telomeres: Measuring Our Chromosomal Age

Tests now can determine the length of your telomeres and give another indirect measure of your biological age. See youngforeverbook.com /resources to learn more about how to test for your biological age. Measuring your telomere length is a good biomarker for how fast you are aging, but in and of itself, it may not be the most important thing to track. However, combining telomere length with DNA methylation, inflammation markers, and other key biomarkers that assess the state of health or function of your core biological systems can provide a robust picture of your biological health and rate of aging. More importantly, telomeres can be monitored and tracked over time to assess the benefits of any lifestyle, supplement, or medication interventions for longevity.

Measuring Your Inflammation Age: The iAge and Systemic Chronic Inflammation Index

Inflammation, as we learned in "Hallmark 10" (Chapter 4), is a core hallmark of aging. In fact, it may be the key driver of all the other hallmarks of aging. But our typical measurements for inflammation, such as C-reactive protein, while in common use, may not be the best markers to assess the inflammation that is correlated with *inflammaging*.

There are literally millions of molecules floating around your bloodstream. Which ones are the most important in assessing your state of health and disease, or your biological age? As part of the 10-year NIH-funded 1000 Immunomes Project, Dr David Furman and his colleagues at Stanford University decided to take an agnostic approach and screened more than 1,000 people from eight to ninety-six years old for about fifty cytokines, most of which are never tested for in conventional medical practice.[5] They called this the *immunome*. Using powerful artificial intelligence technology, they were able to correlate a few inflammatory markers that were more predictive of death and disease than the usual biomarkers doctors use, such as cholesterol, blood pressure, and blood sugar.

They have made this panel of blood inflammatory markers commercially available. It is called the *iAge test,* or inflammatory age test. This new metric predicts multiple chronic diseases and measures the decline of your immune function with aging. The good news is that this measurement of immune dysfunction and inflammation can be reversed through diet, lifestyle, supplements, and even medications and can be tracked over time. They developed two key metrics to assess level of inflammation and immune system age.

- **Systemic Chronic Inflammation Index (SCI Index)**—derived by comparing immune protein levels to those of people with the same chronological age from the 1000 Immunomes Project at Stanford University.
- **Inflammatory clock of aging (iAge)**—showing how much older or younger a person appears with respect to their chronological age.

Function Health offers the iAge and Systemic Chronic Inflammation Index tests too.

Detecting Early Cancer: The Galleri Test, a Liquid Biopsy from Blood

Most of us have heard about the typical cancer screenings, such as mammograms for breast cancer, colonoscopies for colon cancer, Pap tests for cervical cancer, and a PSA test for prostate cancer. These are important tests that can often detect early-stage cancers when they are most curable. But more than 70 percent of cancer deaths are caused by cancers with no recommended screening tests. Until now. Using advanced technologies such as next-generation gene sequencing (for cancer DNA) and machine learning, scientists have been able to find fragments of DNA, called cell-free DNA, from more than fifty cancers in the blood well before any symptoms occur. The test measures DNA methylation patterns that are specific to each individual cancer. If cancers are detected early, more than 90 percent are curable.[6]

This testing is now commercially available. It is called the Galleri test. It does not detect all cancers and should be used in conjunction with regular cancer-screening tests. It is not perfect but is very specific—it will not show a positive result if there is no cancer. And it can pick up about 76 percent of the fifty-plus cancers screened. The cancers that the Galleri test looks for account for 63 percent of all cancer deaths. The Galleri test tells you what the cancer is and where it comes from, and guides follow-up diagnostic testing. While these types of tests will improve over time, this is a powerful way to screen for early cancers that could otherwise prove lethal. An annual test from Function Health is a good insurance policy against dying from cancer.

Total-Body MRI: Looking under the Hood

Innovations in imaging are also helping us detect cancers and disease at very early, curable stages. While we have not quite arrived at the *Star Trek* doctor's capacity to use a tricorder to diagnose everything going on in the human body, we are getting closer. While traditional health care has yet to catch up with the demand for individuals to know and own their health data and order their own tests, many companies are emerging that allow consumers to dive deep into their health with self-care diagnostic tests previously only available through a doctor.

I had the chance to do a full-body MRI scan to look for early cancers, aneurysms, and more. It was a remarkable experience that, while expensive at the time, helped give me a sense of relief about cancer, since both my sister and my father died from malignancies. Companies such as Fountain Life offer full-body MRI scans. Prices are expected to drop from $2,500 to $300 (£2,100 to £252) a scan over the next few years, making regular checkups commonplace.

These newer MRI machines take up to ten times as many images with much higher resolution than standard MRI machines. The scans can detect more than 500 different conditions. A friend recently died from a brain aneurysm at fifty years old, a totally preventable death had he had an MRI scan. While out of reach for most now, full-body MRIs will soon become standard of care and will save billions of dollars in health care costs from preventable cancer deaths and other conditions. Some say they don't want to know what's going on, afraid some dreaded incurable disease will be found, but the advances in medical science, systems medicine, and longevity science will allow us to treat, reverse, and often cure what we may find on the scans. Better to know than to pretend all is well.

A New Type of Heart Checkup: The Cleerly Heart Scan

What is the first symptom for 50 percent of people who have a heart attack? Sudden death. For decades now, doctors have tried to assess heart disease risk by measuring indirect or surrogate makers such as cholesterol and using screening tests such as the cardiac stress test. These tests unfortunately don't tell you how much damage (if any) has been done to the arteries in the heart or determine your personal future risk of a heart attack.

Some doctors have used coronary calcium screening to look for calcified plaque, which is helpful but doesn't accurately predict who will have a heart attack. Other than an angiogram or a more advanced version called an intravascular ultrasound, an invasive, very expensive procedure, we have not been able to look closely at the type of plaque in the arteries.

Is it unstable or stable plaque? Unstable plaque is called *soft plaque* and is more likely to cause a heart attack even without significant narrowing of the arteries. Up to 75 percent of the lesions that cause heart attacks cause only mild narrowing of the arteries and are missed on conventional cardiac stress tests.

Combining new artificial intelligence tools with high-resolution CT scans, Cleerly has created a way of assessing soft plaque. Unstable soft plaque can be turned into calcified stable plaque through lifestyle and medical therapies, and this reduces the risk of heart attacks. These scans are now increasingly available around the country, and forward-thinking cardiologists are using them as the best screening test for heart disease. They must be ordered by your doctor.

Now that we have learned how to map out our biology through the quizzes and testing, let's dive into how to optimize our health and extend our life with the Young Forever Program, starting with the most important pillar: food!

Chapter 14

The Young Forever Longevity Diet: Food as Medicine

When diet is wrong, medicine is of no use. When diet is correct, medicine is of no need.

— AYURVEDIC PROVERB

The most powerful medicine is at the end of your fork, not at the bottom of your pill bottle. Food is more powerful than anything you will find in your medicine cabinet.

— DR MARK HYMAN

As a physician practicing nutritional and functional medicine for 30 years on real patients, using food as medicine, I am humbled by the diversity of human biology and the need to personalize nutritional recommendations. However, a few universal principles exist that can guide the right diet for you.

1. Focus on *quality*.
2. Make *food as medicine* the guiding principle for everything you eat.
3. *Personalize* your diet to fit your metabolism, genetics, and preferences (see Chapter 17).

THE YOUNG FOREVER LONGEVITY DIET

I have jokingly called the diet I recommend the Pegan Diet, poking fun at the diet wars after being on a panel at a conference with a paleo doctor and a vegan cardiologist who were fighting. I said, "If you are vegan and you are paleo, then I must be Pegan." Upon reflection I realized that paleo and vegan diets are identical except for where to get protein (animals or grains and beans). The Pegan Diet is an inclusive, flexible frame that is built on the principles of quality, food is medicine, and personalization. It is designed to be low glycemic (low in starch and sugar), rich in good fats, anti-inflammatory, detoxifying, hormone balancing, energy boosting, and gut healing. It is nutrient dense and rich in longevity phytochemicals, polyphenols, antioxidants, and microbiome-healing fibers. It is designed to regenerate both human and planetary health, which are inseparable.

What to Eat

- **Eat lots of plants.** About three-quarters of your plate should be covered with veggies. Aim for deep colors. Stick with mostly non-starchy veggies. Winter squashes and sweet potatoes are fine in moderation. Choose organic and regenerative when possible. Use the Dirty Dozen and the alternative guides by the PAN (Pesticide Action Network) to choose the least contaminated fruits and vegetables and save money.
- **Lighten up on fruits.** Low-glycemic fruits are best, so stick with berries, kiwis, and watermelon. Enjoy sweeter fruits only occasionally, such as grapes, melons, and higher-glycemic-index fruits. Always eat the whole fruit and avoid fruit juices. Think of dried fruit as candy and keep it to a minimum. When in doubt, get a continuous glucose monitor to track your body's response to different fruits.
- **Load up on foods with healthy fats.** Whole foods such as nuts, seeds, olive oil, avocados, pasture-raised eggs, and small wild fatty fish such as sardines, mackerel, herring, anchovies, and wild salmon contain good fats. For oils, use extra virgin olive oil (at low or no heat), avocado oil (for higher-heat cooking), and organic virgin

coconut oil. (See "Pegan Fats" on page 224 for an explanation of why some fats may not be a good fit for everyone.)

- **Add nuts and seeds.** They help with weight loss, diabetes, and heart disease and provide minerals, protein, good fats, fiber, and more. Almonds, walnuts, pecans, hazelnuts, macadamia nuts, and pumpkin, hemp, chia, and sesame seeds are all great.

- **Think of meat and animal products as condiments** or, as I like to call them, "condi-meats"—not as a main course (which should be colorful vegetables). Servings should be palm-sized. Plant-based meals are fine as long as the protein comes from whole foods, not processed powders, bars, or fake meat. However, to get adequate protein for muscle synthesis as you age, you will need to supplement with animal protein and/or amino acid supplements or vegan protein powders with added amino acids.

- **Buy animal products that have been regeneratively raised, grass-fed, or organic** when possible. They are nutritionally better for you and they are better for the planet. They are also rich in phytonutrients from all the wild and diverse plants the animals consume.

- **Choose pasture-raised eggs.** They are an affordable source of protein and vitamins—including B_{12}, which you can't get from a vegan diet—minerals, antioxidants, and more.

- **Eat fish that is low in mercury and toxins, high in good fats, and wild-caught or sustainably raised.** Sardines, herring, anchovies, mackerel, and salmon all have high omega-3 and low mercury levels. Check out Clean Fish (cleanfish.com) or the Marine Stewardship Council (msc.org/uk) for those that are sustainably harvested/raised and low in toxins.

- **Eat only whole grains (not whole-grain flours) and avoid gluten, especially from American dwarf wheat.** Since all grains boost blood sugar, only eat 60 to 100 grams per day, and choose low-glycemic, gluten-free grains like black rice, quinoa, teff, buckwheat, or amaranth. Try heirloom grains like Himalayan Tartary buckwheat or ancient forms of wheat like einkorn, emmer, or farro.

- **Eat beans.** Lentils are best. Stay away from big starchy beans as staples. Beans contain fiber, protein, and minerals, but some people don't digest them well, and the lectins and phytates in beans can inhibit mineral and protein absorption. If you digest beans without a problem, then up to 75 grams a day is okay.

■ **Avoid sugar** and other foods that spike blood sugar and insulin, such as flour, refined starches, and carbohydrates. Treat sugar in any form as an occasional treat. Your body can't tell the difference between a bagel and a bowl of sugar once it gets below your neck. Liquid sugar calories (from fizzy drinks, energy drinks, sweetened teas, even fruit juice, etc.) cause increased hunger, obesity, and death. Stay away.

■ **Eliminate most grain, bean, and seed oils.** That includes rapeseed, sunflower, grapeseed, and especially corn and soybean oil. Small amounts of expeller or cold-pressed nut and seed oils like sesame, macadamia, and walnut oils are fine to use as condiments or for flavoring. Avocado oil is great for higher-temperature cooking.

■ **Avoid or limit dairy.** Conventional dairy is bad for the environment and most people don't digest it well. Dairy has been linked to inflammation, cancer, osteoporosis, autoimmune conditions, allergic disorders, digestive problems, and more. I recommend avoiding it, except for the occasional grass-fed dairy from yogurt, kefir, grass-fed butter, ghee, and even cheese if it doesn't cause problems for you. Try goat or sheep products instead because they are raised on grass and their milk contains A2 casein, which is less likely to cause inflammation and digestive problems. And always go organic, grass-fed, and ideally regenerative. Some companies now produce regeneratively raised A2 cows' milk, which may be better tolerated. Some nut milks are fine, but watch for added sugar, gut-damaging thickeners, and higher-glycemic oat milks (which also contain gluten). Make your own from nuts soaked in water.

■ **Reduce foods that have been contaminated with pesticides, herbicides, antibiotics, and hormones, and ideally avoid GMO foods.** Look for foods raised or grown in regenerative ways (good for the Earth and for humans), if possible. Check labels for chemicals, additives, preservatives, dyes, artificial sweeteners, or other nonfood ingredients. If you wouldn't find it in your kitchen for cooking, you shouldn't eat it.

Dr Hyman's Pegan Food Pyramid

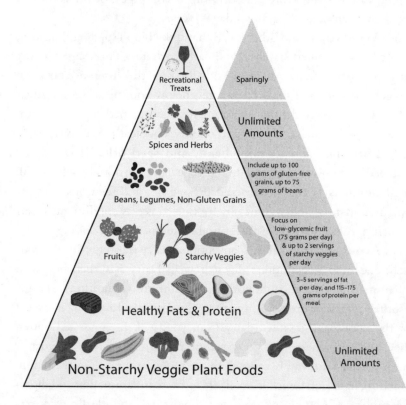

Pegan Fats

There is a subset of people who experience an adverse reaction to saturated fats. We call these people lean mass hyper-responders (LMHR). They typically have an athletic, lean build, are very physically active, and eat a low-carbohydrate, high-fat diet. When they eat a lot of saturated fats, unusual cholesterol patterns can occur.[1] These surprising patterns may be concerning, and individuals need to be monitored for the lipid particle size and number. I created a special "Pegan Fats" list because LMHRs may need to skip certain fats that for others can be healthy.

To help determine if you fit into this category, check out Cholesterol Code (cholesterolcode.com) for more information. You can also ask your doctor to run an NMR or Cardio IQ lipid test or get the Young Forever Function Health Panel to get a deeper dive into your lipid levels and risks. I also find that listening to your body is key. Some people feel amazing consuming coconut oil and other saturated fats, whereas others find they need to stick to fats like avocado and olive oil. Your body is your smartest doctor.

Pegan Fats

Enjoy	Enjoy if not LMHR	Eliminate
Organic extra virgin olive oil	Butter from pastured, grass-fed cows or goats	Vegetable oil
Organic avocado oil	Grass-fed ghee	Soybean oil
Walnut oil	Organic, humanely raised tallow, lard, duck fat, or chicken fat	Rapeseed oil
Almond oil		Corn oil
Macadamia oil		Grapeseed oil
Unrefined sesame oil	Coconut oil or MCT (medium-chain triglyceride) oil	Safflower oil
Tahini		Sunflower oil
Flax oil	Sustainable palm oil (look for Certified Sustainable Palm Oil)	Groundnut oil
Hemp oil		Vegetable shortening
Avocado, olives, and other plant sources of fat		Margarine and butter substitutes
Nuts and seeds		Anything that says "hydrogenated" or "partially hydrogenated"
		Anything fried

Longevity Superfoods: The Power of Phytochemicals

My Young Forever Longevity Diet is about eating the foods that give you vitality, nutrients, and nourishment and skipping the foods that don't. When it comes to longevity, there are some superstar foods that really shine. Want to feel young at any age? Eat these phytonutrients often:

Phytonutrient Category	Source	Benefit
Lutein and zeaxanthin	Cooked spinach Kale Turnip greens Dandelion greens Spring greens Mustard greens	Antioxidant Anti-inflammatory Selectively taken up by the macula Vision health Filters blue light[2]
Lycopene	Tomatoes Watermelon	Cancer prevention Nrf2 activation Anti-inflammatory[3]
α-carotene and β-carotene	Orange, red, and yellow pigmented plants, especially: Carrots Pumpkin Sweet potatoes Cooked spinach Papaya	Antioxidant Cancer prevention Cardioprotective[4]
Curcumin	Turmeric	Anti-inflammatory Neuroprotective Antitumor Antioxidant Nrf2 activation Glutathione biosynthesis[5]
Isothiocyanate	Cruciferous vegetables, especially: Brussels sprouts Garden cress Mustard greens Kale Turnip	Anticancer Anti-inflammatory Antioxidant[6]
Sulforaphane / glucoraphanin	Broccoli sprouts Broccoli	Anticancer Anti-inflammatory Antioxidant Antiaging[7]
Indole-3-carbinol	Cruciferous vegetables, especially: Brussels sprouts Garden cress Mustard greens Kale Turnip	Anticancer

Phytonutrient Category	Source	Benefit
Anthocyanins	Blue-, red-, purple-pigmented plants, especially: Blueberries Black raspberries Purple potatoes Blackberries Cherries Currants	Anticancer Antioxidant Antidiabetic Cardioprotective Vision health Neuroprotective[8]
Flavanols (catechins, epigallocatechin gallate [EGCG])	Black tea Green tea Oolong White tea Dark chocolate	Antioxidant Antiaging Anticancer Repair DNA damage Cardioprotective[9]
Flavanols (quercetin, fisetin, rutin, kaempferol)	Onion Spinach Dill Kale Rocket Watercress Black-eyed peas Chillies Strawberries Apples	Antioxidant Anticancer Activates AMPK Inhibits mTOR Glutathione biosynthesis[10]
Flavones (apigenin)	Parsley Celery Onions Oranges Chamomile Thyme Oregano Basil Herbal teas	Anti-inflammatory Cognitive support Antidiabetic Anticancer[11]
Flavanones (hesperidin)	Lemons Oranges	Antioxidant Anti-inflammatory Neuroprotective Enhances the Nrf2 pathway[12]
Isoflavones (genistein)	Soybeans Tofu Natto Legumes	Antioxidant Anti-inflammatory Anticancer[13]

Phytonutrient Category	Source	Benefit
5-O-caffeoylquinic acid	Coffee	Antioxidant Antidiabetic Cognitive support Detoxification
Resveratrol	Berries Red grapes Blueberries Red wine	Antioxidant Anticancer Cardioprotective Activates AMPK Protects against AGEs[14]
Benzoic acid and cinnamic acid	Mushrooms, especially: Cordyceps Reishi Oyster mushrooms Shiitake Lion's mane Maitake Chaga Agaricus blazei Murrill Antrodia cinnamomea (AC)	Antioxidant Activates Nrf2 pathway Activates sirtuins Protect mitochondria Anticancer Antidiabetic[15]
Oleuropein	Olives Olive oil	Anticancer Antioxidant Cardioprotective Anti-inflammatory Neuroprotective[16]
Omega-3 fatty acids Docosahexaenoic acid (DHA) and eicosapentaenoic acid (EPA)	Algae Fish that feed on algae, especially: Fatty fish Salmon Sardines Fish oil Fish eggs Krill Krill oil	Anti-inflammatory Cardioprotective Cognitive support
Lauric acid	Unrefined coconut oil MCT oil	Anti-inflammatory Microbiome support Neuroprotective[17]
Caprylic acid	Unrefined coconut oil MCT oil Palm oil (only Certified Sustainable Palm Oil)	Anti-inflammatory Neuroprotective Cardioprotective Blood sugar balance[18]

Calorie Restriction Mimetics: Hacking Starvation

The one thing proven in longevity science is that eating fewer calories and triggering the starvation response in the body has significant long-term benefits on health and longevity.[19] But in the search for ways to hack calorie restriction long term without being miserable and hungry, losing muscle and bone density, reducing sex hormones and libido, and slowing wound healing, scientists have found many roads to Rome.

Luckily, there are ways to mimic calorie restriction without starving yourself. Here are several listed in order of the simplest and easiest to implement to more advanced strategies for activating your longevity pathways. You can start with time-restricted eating and experiment with other options that speak to you.

1. **Time-restricted eating** narrows the eating window to 8 to 12 hours. You can do this daily or three or four times a week depending on your health and weight. For example, you can finish dinner at 7 p.m. and have breakfast at 9 a.m. (a 14-hour fast). There should be at least 12 hours a day of not eating between dinner and breakfast.

2. **Intermittent fasts** of 24 to 36 hours or even fasts of three days to a week periodically are another option. Even a weekly 24-hour fast can trigger a deep cleaning.

3. **Fasting-mimicking diets.** Valter Longo, a leading longevity researcher at the University of Southern California, has developed a fasting-mimicking diet[20] shown to be effective in extending life in animal models, and in weight loss, improving insulin resistance, cholesterol, dementia, autoimmunity, and response to chemotherapy and radiation in cancer patients.[21] It is a plant-based diet of 800 calories per day for five days and can be done monthly or quarterly. You can learn more at the website for ProLon FMD (prolonfmd.com).

4. **Ketogenic diet.** Another potential way to activate your longevity pathways is through a ketogenic diet: 70 to 75 percent fat, 20 to 25 percent protein, and 5 percent carbohydrates. For those who have

severe metabolic disease, such as type 2 diabetes, a longer-term ketogenic diet has completely reversed type 2 diabetes in 60 percent of people and has gotten 90 to 100 percent off medication and insulin. For people with insulin resistance (about nine in ten Americans), a short- or longer-term ketogenic diet can quickly reverse metabolic dysfunction and improve your cholesterol profile. Then, transitioning to the Young Forever Longevity Diet for the long term can keep you healthy.

DR HYMAN'S HEALTHY AGING SHAKE

This shake is great for breakfast after a 12- to 16-hour fast, or drink it within an hour of exercise, especially strength training. It provides support for muscle synthesis, mitochondrial health and repair, microbiome support, detoxification support, and hormone and adrenal support, and it includes compounds that support healthy aging. It keeps me balanced and energetic. The key is to get the right amount and quality of protein after your workout (usually 30 grams of animal protein or vegan proteins supplemented with branched-chain amino acids needed for muscle synthesis). I use regeneratively raised goat whey because it is cleanest and easiest to use. The rest of the ingredients are optional, but include as many as you can.

Prep Time: 5 minutes

Serves: 1 to 2

Ingredients:

30 grams (2 scoops) goat whey from organic or regeneratively raised goats (Mt. Capra and Naked Goat are good brands); or, if vegan, 42 grams (2 scoops) Garden of Life Sport Organic Plant-Based Protein (with added branched-chain amino acids for protein synthesis)

1 packet Mitopure (from pomegranate) for mitophagy and muscle building from Timeline Nutrition

5 grams (1 scoop) creatine by Thorne for muscle synthesis

9 grams (1 scoop) Gut Food by Farmacy for gut healing and support; Gut Food contains extensively researched probiotics, prebiotics, and polyphenols, like a multivitamin for the gut. You can find it at gutfood.com (soon to be available in the UK) .

1 tablespoon MCT oil or Brain Octane oil (for energy, brain function)

1 teaspoon Stamets 7 Mushroom Powder (for energy, immunity, and stress resilience; 7 Mushroom Powder is an adaptogenic mushroom powder that includes reishi, chaga, lion's mane, cordyceps, and more)

240 to 360 ml unsweetened macadamia milk or other nut or seed milk without emulsifiers or sweeteners (I recommend Elmhurst)

1 handful frozen berries

Additional options:

1 scoop or packet Athletic Greens (greens powder with vitamins and minerals)

1 tablespoon each Organic Pomegranate and Cranberry Concentrate (polyphenols for healthy microbiome support)

1 teaspoon matcha powder by Navitas (green tea with epigallocatechin gallate [EGCG], which supports the growth of a healthy microbiome)

Directions:

In a blender, combine all the ingredients. Blend until smooth; drink, and enjoy feeling more youthful.

In addition to these approaches, science has discovered promising compounds that mimic calorie restriction, including resveratrol, the flavonols quercetin, myricetin, kaempferol, butein, fisetin from strawberries, hesperidin, piceatannol from rhubarb, epigallocatechins from green tea, polyphenols from apples, black rice extracts, blueberry extracts, proanthocyanidins in persimmon, tannic acid (TA), gallic acid (GA) and ellagic acid (EA), curcumin, and omega-3 fats.[22] And surely we will discover more. We can eat our way to longevity boosted by a few supplements containing these compounds. These phyto-chemicals are found in many foods, spices, and drinks, such as apples, onions, green tea, rhubarb, persimmons, blueberries, black rice, green tea, red grapes, Himalayan Tartary buckwheat, turmeric, and sardines.

They may help us regulate our longevity switches without having to restrict calories. However, using the simple strategies of time-restricted eating and intermittent fasts combined with phytochemicals can be a great place to start.

The foundation of health and longevity is diet. You can exercise and meditate and sleep and take all the supplements in the world, but unless you focus on high-quality, nutrient-dense, whole foods person-alized to your own needs and preferences, you will not achieve health or longevity. Focus on food as medicine. Upgrade your diet and bio-logical software with each bite. Your fork is the most powerful tool you have to change your health and your life. Use it wisely.

Chapter 15

The Young Forever Supplements for Longevity

Science has proven that while your genes control your biology, a rather simple, nondrug formula of nutrient-rich food, targeted supplements to address missing precursors and lifestyle changes can keep your genes in perpetual "repair" mode.

—DR SARA GOTTFRIED

The topic of nutritional and herbal supplements is fraught with confusion, misinformation, incomplete research, and conflicting data. Add to that the inadequate regulation for quality standards in manufacturing, or for purity and potency, and choosing supplements is a potential minefield.

The long-standing debate about the need for nutritional supplements if you eat a "balanced diet" surely will continue. Many doctors still believe that vitamins just make expensive urine. If that were true, we should stop drinking water because we pee it out! Clearly, we use what we need and excrete the rest. In fact, other than in deficiency diseases like scurvy or rickets, most people don't understand the role of nutrients in our basic biochemical processes. Trillions and trillions of chemical reactions occur in your body every second. Every single one requires a helper or an enzyme, and each enzyme requires its own helper or coenzyme. Vitamins and minerals are the coenzymes essential to grease the wheels of our vast metabolic pathways.

Dr Robert Heaney, the grandfather of vitamin D research, described what he termed *long-latency deficiency disease.*[1] If you have an acute deficiency of vitamin D, you get rickets. Long-term low-level deficiency or insufficiency can cause osteoporosis, cancer, depression, muscle weakness, heart disease, and dementia. The current RDAs (recommended dietary allowances) are the *minimum* amount of vitamins you need to avoid a deficiency disease, not the amount required for optimal health. How much vitamin D do you need to prevent rickets? About 30 units a day. How much do you need for optimal health? Around 2,000 to 5,000 units of vitamin D_3 a day. The same is true for most nutrients.

After having tested nutritional status on 10,000 patients over 30 years, and mostly in a health-conscious population, I can assure you that nutritional deficiencies are rampant. According to the NHANES government nutritional study, more than 90 percent of Americans are deficient in one or more nutrients at the RDA level.[2] It's hard to believe, but 10 percent of Americans are deficient in vitamin C and actually have scurvy. More than 90 percent are deficient in omega-3 fats, 80 percent are low in vitamin D, and 45 percent are deficient in magnesium and iron, with folate and zinc not far behind. Lack of these nutrients moves us rapidly down the trajectory of disease and aging.

You may wonder why we need vitamins now if humans evolved for 200,000 years without supplements. If you lived like our ancestors and hunted and gathered your own wild food, including mushrooms and 800 different species of wild plants rich in omega-3 fats, phytonutrients, vitamins, and minerals; if you ate offal, bone marrow, and wild fish; if you spent your days half-clothed outside in the sun; and if you were never exposed to environmental toxins or chronic stress and slept 8 to 9 hours a night, waking and sleeping with the sun — then, no, you would not need nutritional supplements. If that describes you, skip the supplements. For the rest of us, supplements are essential insurance against our nutrient-depleted diet, toxic environment, and high-stress lives.

I think of nutritional supplements in two ways: first, as the foundational nutrients everyone needs for life; second, as specifically targeted supplements based on your unique needs (genetics, age, lifestyle, testing, and imbalances in the core biological networks or systems). A good multivitamin and mineral, vitamin D_3, omega-3 fats, magnesium, and support for methylation (special forms of folate, B_6 and B_{12}, and other methylation nutrients) are essential for everyone. And given our gut-busting life, a good probiotic is also important. Not all supplements are created equal. They are unregulated, so it is critical to choose supplements that undergo rigorous manufacturing according to good manufacturing practices and independent / third-party testing for purity and potency, contain the most bioavailable and active forms of nutrients, and are free of fillers, additive, dyes, and preservatives. Do you really need a vitamin made with blue dye?

At youngforeverbook.com/resources, I provide a complete list of the specific products and brands and doses I recommend. The companies I use most with my patients include Pure Encapsulations, Xymogen, Designs for Health, Metagenics, Big Bold Health, Thorne, and Natural Factors.

LONGEVITY SUPPLEMENT SUPPORT: THE CORE PLAN

In this core plan I list my recommended supplements and favorite brands and products. There are equivalent brands available, and you will find more options at youngforeverbook.com/resources. These should be foundational for everyone. For those of you who want to upgrade your supplement plan, you can add the Advanced Longevity Support Supplements, on page 236, which have the most data for activating longevity pathways. Additional Nutritional Support, on page 239, may be added to optimize mitochondrial function.

Core Supplement Plan

■ **Vitamin D_3, 2,000 to 5,000 IU a day** with vitamin K_2 (including MK-7 form), such as Vitamin D Supreme by Designs for Health.

- **EPA/DHA (omega-3 supplements), 1 to 2 grams a day.**
Dutch Harbor Omega from Big Bold Health is cold processed, which
prevents oxidation of the fats and preserves active anti-inflammatory
compounds called *resolvins;* take 2 softgels a day.
- **Multivitamin and mineral.** Getting a complete array of all the
micronutrient vitamins and minerals is important to optimizing your
metabolic functioning. This should include all the B vitamins in the correct forms for methylation, such as 5 methyl-folate instead of folate,
or methylcobalamin instead of hydroxycobalamin, or pyridoxal-5-
phosphate instead of B_6. I recommend Multi t/d, 2 a day, by Pure Encapsulations or Polyphenol Nutrients by Pure Encapsulations; take 3 per day.
- **Additional methylation support.** You may need extra support
for methylation if a high homocysteine level (over 10 mcmol/L) is indicated on your Young Forever Function Health Panel. For extra methylation support I recommend Homocysteine Supreme by Designs for
Health; take 2 per day.
- **Magnesium glycinate or citrate, 200 to 600 mg a day** to
support sleep, relaxation, and muscle function (45 percent are deficient in
magnesium).[3] I recommend magnesium glycinate for those who do not
have constipation and magnesium citrate if you tend to be constipated.
Both are available from Pure Encapsulations; take 2 to 4 capsules a day.
- **Probiotics** to support a healthy microbiome. Probiotic 50B by
Pure Encapsulations is a good basic probiotic; take 1 a day. Some people
may need more specialized probiotics depending on their unique needs.

ADVANCED LONGEVITY SUPPORT SUPPLEMENTS

These compounds are safe, effective, supported by research, and work
on various pathways that promote longevity, including mTOR, AMPK,
insulin signaling, sirtuins, and inflammation and antioxidant systems,
and as senolytics (compounds that kill inflammation-producing zombie cells). Many of these compounds work on multiple pathways. For
example, fisetin, resveratrol, and quercetin are all sirtuin activators.
Nrf2 activators regulate our master antioxidant systems, including

glutathione, and optimize mitochondrial function. But they also support detoxification and reduce inflammation. Those Nrf2 activators include sulforaphane (an extract from broccoli), pterostilbene (a more bioavailable form of resveratrol found in berries, almonds, and grapes), curcumin, and green tea extract (EGCG), among others.

Following is the advanced longevity stack I recommend daily. I've listed basic supplement ranges. You may need higher or lower doses, depending on your age, health status, and genetics, so ideally work with a functional medicine practitioner to determine your current levels and recommended dosage.

- **NMN or NR, 1,000 mg a day** to support NAD+ production and function. MIB-626, developed by Metro International Biotech, is pharmaceutical-grade NMN that is in clinical trials now; it may be more effective than other preparations.[4] NMN by Renue by Science offers NMN products that are available now. Other companies have different forms of NAD+-boosting compounds. Tru Niagen and NAD3, a nutraceutical from *Wasabia japonica* available in some supplements, are also being used to boost NAD+. NAD+ may also be given subcutaneously (usually 100 mg a day) or intravenously, often at doses of 500 mg. More research is needed to determine the best form and route of administration. There is some early evidence from animal models that NAD+ may fuel the growth of some cancers in a test tube. If you have cancer I would hold off on this therapy until more data is available.

- **Fisetin, 500 to 1,000 mg a day** from strawberries, apples, and persimmons, is the flavonoid with the most potent senolytic effects, and it also stimulates autophagy and activates sirtuins and AMPK.[5] It may be more effective than the combination of quercetin and dastinib (a chemotherapy drug) in reversing biological age. Senolytic Synergy by Designs for Health contains a blend of phytochemicals, including curcumin, quercetin, red grape powder, fisetin, and ginseng; take 2 capsules twice a day.

- **Quercetin and other flavonols.** HTB Rejuvenate by Big Bold Health contains high levels of quercetin, luteolin, hesperidin, and other bioflavonoids to support healthy immune function and longevity. It is made from Himalayan Tartary buckwheat. Take 2 daily or 2 twice daily for optimal dose. It is unique in its effects on immune rejuvenation and is a staple for me.

- **Pterostilbene, 100 mg once or twice a day.** This is more effective than resveratrol as a sirtuin activator.[6] PolyResveratrol-SR by Thorne is a good combination of pterostilbene, quercetin, curcumin, and EGCG; take 2 twice a day.

- **Curcumin, 500 to 1,000 mg a day** from the spice turmeric. It is activated by black pepper, which is often added to curcumin formulations. Curcumin with bioperine (from black pepper) by Pure Encapsulations is a good source; take 1 to 2 capsules twice a day.

- **Epigallocatechin gallate (EGCG), 500 to 1,000 mg a day** from green tea. This can be taken in combination with other nutrients (as in PolyResveratrol-SR), or as a single ingredient in EGCG by Designs for Health; take 1 to 2 capsules a day.

- **Glucoraphanin,** which converts to sulforaphane in the body, from broccoli-seed extract, is a powerful detoxifier, antioxidant, and modulator of gene expression. A well-researched brand is Xymogen's OncoPLEX; take 30 mg twice a day.

- **Urolithin A** is available as Mitopure from Timeline Nutrition. Take 1 packet or 2 capsules a day.

Sarcopenia Support

- **Branched-chain amino acids** (leucine, isoleucine, valine) are essential for muscle synthesis.[7] Amino Acid Complex from Thorne (1 scoop a day between meals) is a well-researched high-leucine blend of all essential amino acids that supports sports, fitness, and training-related activities and promotes the growth of muscle mass in individuals who need to preserve it, including the elderly. This is an especially important supplement for vegans. You can also take BCAA by Pure Encapsulations, 3,000 mg or 1 scoop a day.

- **Creatine, 5 to 10 grams daily,** increases muscle synthesis and mitochondrial function in combination with exercise and strength training.[8] You can take Creatine by Thorne; take 5 grams (1 scoop) to 10 grams (2 scoops) daily.

ADDITIONAL NUTRITIONAL SUPPORT

Depending on your health status, goals, and willingness to up your nutritional support, the following are supplements that are important for mitochondrial function, energy production, detoxification, and reducing inflammation. You can take them together or individually:

■ **RegenerLife by Natural Factors, 1 scoop or 4 capsules a day,** includes the targeted nutrients acetyl-L-carnitine, coenzyme Q10, L-glutathione, superoxide dismutase, and a specialized ATP formula, which supports mitochondrial function and reduces oxidative stress and inflammation.

■ **Acetyl-L-carnitine, 500 to 1,000 mg a day,** supports mitochondrial function.

■ **N-acetylcysteine, 600 mg twice a day,** supports glutathione production.

■ **PQQ, a derivative of coenzyme Q10, 100 to 200 mg a day,** aids mitochondrial function.

■ **Alpha-lipoic acid, 300 to 600 mg a day,** an antioxidant and detoxifier, supports insulin sensitivity and glucose control. ALAmax CR by Xymogen (600 mg a day) is the brand I recommend.

Butein: A Promising Longevity Phytochemical

Butein has a wide range of biological properties, including antioxidant, anti-inflammatory, anticancer, antidiabetic, hypotensive, and neuroprotective effects. It has been shown to affect multiple molecular targets, including the master transcription factor nuclear factor-κB (NfKB), which is the main driver of inflammation.[9] It will soon likely be available as a supplement.

MEDICATIONS FOR LONGEVITY: WORKS IN PROGRESS

The longevity drug pipeline is accelerating fast. Billions of dollars are spent on research looking for drugs that optimize the longevity pathways, such as mTOR, AMPK, and sirtuins, or that act as senolytics. Although the Young Forever Program uses diet, lifestyle, and hormesis, along with nutrients and phytochemicals, to do the same things as, and often better than, most drugs, there may be a place for existing or new medications that can optimize health and aging. I do not recommend you take these medications until we have more data or upon consultation with your doctor.

■ **Metformin, 500 mg twice a day,** before lunch and dinner is a common regimen used by those experimenting with its longevity benefits (see Chapter 4). The TAME Trial will soon reveal how effective it is; however, to date, lifestyle interventions have been far more effective than metformin in addressing insulin resistance.

■ **Rapamycin, 2 mg three times a week, cycling 5 weeks on and 8 weeks off,** is one regimen used by longevity enthusiasts, but it still requires far more research to determine the safest, most effective dose and schedule (see Chapter 4). Longevity hackers are experimenting with a variety of dosing and timing regimens. Rapalogs, or analogs of rapamycin, may turn out to be as or more effective with potentially fewer side effects. In mice, rapamycin increases middle-age life expectancy by 60 percent and reverses every age-related dysfunction. That's pretty exciting data and needs to be replicated in humans.

While diet is the foundation of the Young Forever Program, judicious use of evidence-based nutritional supplements can be a powerful boost to your health and well-being. And research is underway on potential medications such as rapamycin and metformin, which may become part of everyone's longevity regimen soon. Next, we jump into the powerful effects of simple lifestyle changes on our health and our life span.

The Young Forever Lifestyle Practices: How to Exercise, De-Stress, Sleep, Find Your Purpose, and Activate Hormesis

The doctor of the future will give no medicine, but will interest his patient in the care of the human frame, in diet and in the cause and prevention of disease.

— THOMAS EDISON

Many simple, inexpensive lifestyle practices help enhance our health and activate our longevity pathways. Learning how to optimize exercise, stress reduction, and sleep is key to achieving a long and healthy life. Exploring ways to find meaning and purpose can help you deepen your connection to yourself, your family, and your work and help you live longer! Adding a few simple hormesis practices on a regular basis can help you keep your body young, strong, and healthy.

EXERCISE: THE FOUNTAIN OF YOUTH

The joke is that if you don't move, you won't. The good news is that you will get the most dramatic gains in health and longevity when you go from doing nothing to doing something, like a 30-minute walk a day. However, if you want to achieve maximum benefits, you must focus on three key aspects of fitness:

1. Aerobic conditioning (to optimize your VO$_2$ max)
2. Strength and muscle mass and function
3. Flexibility and agility

Thankfully there are so many options for keeping the body moving, and some of them are more like play than what you think of as exercising. Think biking, swimming, dancing, skiing, and tennis, for instance.

What is essential?

Aerobic Conditioning

If you don't exercise at all, just start walking.

If you want to optimize your VO$_2$ max and fitness, then do more vigorous exercise three or more days a week, such as jogging, biking, tennis, dancing, rowing, or using a treadmill or elliptical machine. This gets your lymphatic system moving.

If you want to optimize even further, start a high-intensity interval training (HIIT) program, where you push yourself to your max capacity, as if you were running from a tiger, for 45 to 60 seconds, followed by a 3-minute slow walk or light jog. Doing a few cycles for 30 minutes three times a week can have dramatic benefits, including increasing your metabolism, losing weight, and boosting your VO$_2$ max.

How to Exercise for Health and Longevity

There are no shortage of programs, apps, and tools to help you start (see youngforeverbook.com/resources) and create healthy habits. Here are some basic starting ideas for getting moving:

- Go for a 20-minute walk first thing in the morning.
- Play a sport. Play catch with your kids, take up Frisbee golf, play pickleball, shoot some hoops.
- Invest in a standing desk, treadmill desk, or under-desk elliptical. Just standing more can reduce your risk of death.[1]
- Pick up an outdoor hobby. Try gardening, landscaping, hiking, bird-watching, photography, fishing, hunting, canoeing, or kayaking.

■ Invite friends to join a group exercise class. Getting healthy is a team sport. Most gyms and fitness facilities offer a range of group classes, from spin classes to Zumba to chair yoga. You're way more likely to stick with an exercise routine if you have an accountability buddy.

■ Have fun! You don't need to visit a gym to incorporate daily movement.

Strength Training

Preserving muscle, building muscle, and optimizing muscle function are the keys to the fountain of youth.[2] How do you do this? Put your muscles to work.

Try weight lifting, resistance bands, and body-weight exercise. I didn't start doing weight training until I was sixty years old because I told myself that biking, tennis, and yoga were good enough. I was wrong. My overall health, muscle mass, balance, agility, and strength, and my back pain (after two surgeries) have dramatically improved. My body is more fit and muscular at sixty-three than it was at twenty, thirty, forty, or fifty. Discover what works for you. Personally I don't love going to the gym. I started a home-training program with TB12 Sports (tb12sports.com), Tom Brady's program of band workouts and pliability. I do 30 minutes of intense band workouts three to four times a week. The bands are a small investment, and an app guides you through a comprehensive workout program. I travel with the bands and use them everywhere. They are less likely to cause injury than weights.

If strength training is new for you, then it's best to work with someone experienced like a trainer, so you learn how to correctly perform the exercises and avoid injury. It is never too late to start. I got my father started at eighty-nine years old because he was having trouble getting out of a chair. What often puts people in nursing homes is sarcopenia and the inability to do the tasks of daily life.

Ideally do three strength-training days each week to build and maintain your muscles and increase your mitochondria, which in turn will increase your energy, fat burning, and longevity.

Flexibility and Agility

Just like the Tin Man from *The Wizard of Oz,* we tend to rust as we age and need some lubrication. Flexibility and agility are key to staying active and pain-free. Yoga is the most effective therapy for helping older adults stay functional and pain-free.[3]

A twelve-week intervention incorporating classical yoga postures, breathing exercises, and meditation was associated with positive changes in the levels of biomarkers of cellular aging including 8–OH2dG, a product of DNA damage; oxidative stress markers; and telomeres. It also improves neural connections, memory, and inflammation. Not bad for a little stretching!

With online yoga classes and yoga studios on nearly every corner, yoga is a simple practice that will help you stay flexible and happy. My favorite is hot yoga, which gives me the quintuple benefit of stretching, strength, aerobic conditioning, stress reduction, and heat therapy.

HEALING OUR MINDS, HEARTS, AND SPIRITS: THE ANTIDOTE TO THE DANGERS OF CHRONIC STRESS

For most of the twentieth and twenty-first centuries, the tools for healing our minds, hearts, and souls have been limited to various models of psychotherapy and psychiatric medication. But now, even top-tier institutions have departments dedicated to the study of how nutrition and metabolic health affect mental health and psychological disorders. These are focused on biological causes that must be addressed, including poor nutrition and nutritional deficiencies, environmental toxins, hormone imbalances, dysbiosis of our microbiome, and inflammatory root causes.

Today, there is a revolution happening in the treatment of mental illness, trauma, and stress that focuses in new ways on the underlying psychological roots of mental health or disease. Gabor Maté, a physician who has dedicated his life to reimagining mental health through the lens of trauma, has helped us rethink our approach to psychological and emotional dysfunction. He suffered abandonment trauma after his mother gave him to a stranger as a baby to protect him from the Nazis near the end of World War II, and he invites us all to look at the traumas we have experienced in our lives, whether big or small. These could be what he calls microtraumas, like not being loved well enough by our parents, being neglected, or living in our stressed-out toxic culture, or macrotraumas, like sexual or physical abuse or worse. In his book *The Myth of Normal: Trauma, Illness, and Healing in a Toxic Culture* he provides a new road map for healing from the traumas that interfere with our ability to live whole and fulfilled lives, not driven by our old conditioning.

In Chapter 17, we will explore emerging treatments for trauma and mental illness using psychedelic therapy. For basic stress management, here are some simple ways to prioritize self-care and reset your stress response.

- Try simple breathing practices such as Take 5: five deep breaths slowly in and out when you wake, before each meal, and at bedtime.
- Learn how to meditate. It has been a game changer for me. Try Ziva Meditation (zivameditation.com) to learn a simple 20-minute practice you can do anywhere.
- Try guided meditations or yoga nidra (yogic sleep) practices daily even for 10 minutes. If you don't have 10 minutes a day, then it's worth taking a hard look at your life!
- Start or continue a regular yoga practice. Even 15 minutes a day of breathing and stretching can reset our nervous system.
- Try forest bathing, or what we used to call taking a walk in the woods!
- Write your deepest feelings and thoughts in a journal daily—it has been proven to lower inflammation and improve overall well-being and health.[4]
- Keep a notebook by your bed and write three different things you're grateful for every day when you wake up. Try not to repeat anything! In his book *Flourish,* Martin Seligman unpacks the science of gratitude and its effects on your health and happiness. It is a simple practice to focus on what's right and good and not on what's wrong or bad.

▪ Build your close friend network. Start an in-person or Zoom support group to create your own safe healing environment and to share your life with all its ups and downs. Being known and seen and loved is the best medicine.

▪ Practice massage with your partner or friend or get a professional massage weekly if you can.

▪ Start an exercise and strength-training routine; not only does exercise release your feel-good neurotransmitters serotonin and dopamine,[5] but resistance training has been shown to help mitigate age-related testosterone decline.[6] It's a form of both self-care and hormone support!

Optimizing Sleep for Longevity

Here's how to restore your natural sleep rhythm. It may take weeks or months, but using these tools in a coordinated way will eventually reset your biological rhythms.

▪ Practice the regular rhythms of sleep. Go to bed and wake up at the same time each day.

▪ Use your bed for sleep and romance only, not reading or television.

▪ Create an aesthetic environment that encourages sleep—use serene and restful colors and eliminate clutter and distraction.

▪ Create total darkness and quiet. Consider using eyeshades and earplugs.

▪ Get grounded. Electromagnetic frequencies can impair sleep. I recommend turning off Wi-Fi and keeping all your electronic devices away from your bed. Create a charging station in a common area of your home and encourage all your family members to "check in" their devices before bed.

▪ Eliminate blue-light exposure for 2 to 3 hours before bed. Avoid computers, smartphones, tablets, and television 2 hours before bed. Avoiding blue-spectrum light after the sun goes down helps your brain reset for sleep and increases melatonin. Ideally use blue-blocker glasses after sunset, a simple hack that pays sleep and health dividends.

■ Avoid caffeine. It may help you stay awake during the day, but it interferes with your sleep.

■ Avoid alcohol. It helps you get to sleep but causes interruptions in sleep and poor-quality sleep, something I have seen firsthand from data on my Oura Ring.

■ Get regular exposure to daylight for at least 20 minutes daily. The light from the sun enters your eyes and triggers your brain to release specific chemicals and hormones like melatonin that are vital to healthy sleep, mood, and aging.

■ Eat no later than 3 hours before bed. Eating a heavy meal prior to bed will lead to a bad night's sleep.

■ Don't exercise vigorously after dinner. It excites the body and makes it more difficult to get to sleep.

■ Write down your worries. One hour before bed, write down the things that are causing you anxiety and make plans for what you might have to do the next day to reduce your worry. It will free up your mind and energy to move into deep and restful sleep.

■ Take a hot Epsom salts and aromatherapy bath with lavender oil. Raising your body temperature before bed helps to induce sleep. A hot bath also relaxes your muscles and reduces physical and psychic tension. By adding 500 grams of Epsom salts (magnesium sulfate) and 10 drops of lavender oil, you will gain the benefits of magnesium absorbed through your skin to relax your muscles as well as the cortisol-lowering effects of lavender.

■ Get a massage or stretch before bed. This helps relax the body, making it easier to fall asleep.

■ Warm your middle. A hot water bottle, heating pad, or warm body can do the trick. This raises your core temperature and helps trigger the proper chemistry for sleep.

■ Avoid medications that interfere with sleep. These include sedatives (these are used to treat insomnia but ultimately lead to dependence and disruption of normal sleep rhythms and architecture), antihistamines, stimulants, cold medication, steroids, and headache medication that contains caffeine (such as Fioricet).

▪ Use herbal therapies. Try 100 to 200 mg of passionflower or 320 to 480 mg of valerian (*Valeriana officinalis*) root extract standardized to 0.2 percent valerenic acid 1 hour before bed.

▪ Take 200 to 400 mg of magnesium citrate or glycinate before bed. Magnesium is a powerful relaxation mineral for the nervous system and muscles.

▪ Try 0.5 to 2 mg of melatonin before bed.

▪ Other supplements and herbs can be helpful in getting some shut-eye. Try calcium, L-theanine (an amino acid from green tea), GABA, 5-HTP, and magnolia.

▪ Find guided relaxation, yoga nidra, meditation, and guided imagery options online and listen to them before bed. Any of these may help you get to sleep.

▪ Try binaural beats sound meditation, which synchronizes brain waves for deep sleep. You can find videos on YouTube. They can be used before bed or in the middle of the night to help you fall back asleep.

▪ Try my free Sleep Master Class available at drhyman.com/sleep.

If after trying these strategies you still struggle with sleep, please see a functional medicine practitioner who can determine whether things like food sensitivities, thyroid problems, menopause, fibromyalgia, chronic fatigue syndrome, heavy metal toxicity, stress, or depression is interfering with your sleep. You can find one at the website of the Institute for Functional Medicine (ifm.org). Consider getting tested for sleep disorders such as sleep apnea. Getting good sleep is essential for your health and longevity.

HOW TO FIND MEANING AND PURPOSE

What are some ways to connect to your purpose?

1. **Develop a growth mindset.** Explore ways to learn and be curious about yourself and the world. Address the parts of yourself and

your life that may not be working, and explore avenues for personal development.

2. **Create a vision statement.** What matters to you? What are your personal goals? What are your dreams?

3. **Practice altruism and serving others.** The same brain circuits that get rewarded with cocaine or heroin are also stimulated by altruism, which is much safer and healthier! Find a cause that matters to you and be part of making the world a better place. A well-known Indian guru, Neem Karoli Baba, had a very simple teaching to reach awakening: Love everyone; serve everyone. And he added: Feed everyone! Volunteer; find ways to give back in your community. Practice random acts of kindness.

4. **Transform your struggles and pain into purpose.** Most of us have had either micro- or macrotraumas in our lives. Using those experiences to help others is a powerful road to well-being and happiness. When I was in my midthirties, I developed chronic fatigue syndrome from mercury poisoning and Lyme disease. I cured myself with functional medicine, and that propelled me to want to help others who suffer needlessly. Through my own pain, I found my life's purpose.

5. **Discover your passions.** Spend time doing things that you love and that give you joy. Take time to uncover your passions, which might be buried under society's expectations of you. We often live our lives based on what we think we *should* do and don't follow or explore our dreams for ourselves. You can reinvent your life at any age. Take time to examine your life and make the changes you need to bring more passion and joy to what you do.

6. **Connect to a community.** The most powerful way to stay healthy and connect to your purpose is to be part of some type of community. It could be a book club or bowling buddies. Those who are connected to others live longer. During COVID, I reached out to my closest male friends to start a men's group. We meet every week for 2 hours on Zoom, and it has deeply enriched my life.

7. **Connect with friends or colleagues who inspire you.** You are only as healthy as the people you spend the most time with. If your

friends are going to yoga and eating healthy, or are focused on growth and personal development, you will be healthier than if your friends are eating junk food and bingeing on Netflix.

8. **Cultivate your mind by reading.** Learn about the world, and about yourself. Read nonfiction and fiction to explore different ways of seeing, being, and knowing that connect you to something greater than yourself.

9. **Learn to love and be kind to yourself.** It's not as easy as it sounds. If we talked to our friends the same way we talk to ourselves, we would find ourselves pretty much alone. Spiritual teacher Ram Dass encourages us to engage in nonjudgmental loving self-awareness. Learn to recognize your negative inner dialogue, or what leading psychiatrist Dr Daniel Amen calls ANTs (automatic negative thoughts), and to let them pass over like a rain cloud.

10. **Take time for self-care.** When you nurture your well-being, you become a source of energy and light for yourself and others. We live in a culture where productivity is valued over things that fill up our hearts and souls. Take time to develop simple practices that bring you back to yourself and support the health of your body and mind and heart.

ACTIVATING HORMESIS: PRACTICES FOR HEALTH AND LONGEVITY

We evolved in a stressful environment that was not carefully thermoregulated to 68°F/20°C, where food was not available everywhere at every hour, where our bodies were forced to move and lift and bend and run to survive. Modern life insulates us from most of the physical hardships experienced by our evolutionary ancestors. Here are some simple ways to safely stress your system so that it becomes stronger, happier, more resilient, and younger.

Calorie-Restriction Hacks

Eating fewer calories or fasting for short periods of time has been proven to extend health span and life span.[7] Refer to Chapter 14 for details on time-restricted eating, intermittent fasting, a fasting-mimicking diet, and a ketogenic diet (which mimics starvation). Start with an overnight fast of 12 to 14 hours, limiting your eating window to 10 to 12 hours. Try the phytochemicals that mimic calorie restriction we reviewed in Chapter 14.

Hack Exercise for Longevity

If there were a longevity pill, it would be exercise. Certain forms of exercise, as we reviewed earlier, are more effective at optimizing our health, metabolism, and longevity. Our aerobic condition, strength, muscle mass, and flexibility and agility are essential for staying healthy and aging well. One main reason why exercise is so effective at keeping us young is due to its hormetic effects. We covered hormesis in detail in Chapter 15, but here are the best practices for activating hormesis through exercise.

1. **Boost your VO_2 max.** This is a measure of your metabolism, mitochondria, and fitness level. The higher it is, the longer you will live.[8] The simple but powerful practice of high-intensity interval training is the best way to boost your VO_2 max.

2. **Maximize muscle.** The currency of healthy aging is muscle—lean, high-performance muscle. There is no way around this, and it takes as little as 30 minutes three times a week. Find what works for you and do it consistently.

3. **Get flexible.** Keeping your muscles, tendons, and ligaments pliable and flexible is key to mobility, agility, balance, and living pain-free as we age. Yoga is the best way to keep your body supple and agile as you age.

Hot and Cold Therapy

Getting out of your thermo-regulated environment provides a powerful stimulus for health and longevity. Cold and hot treatments are available at low or no cost to almost everyone. For cold immersion, add breath work, such as Wim Hof's breathing technique, to help you adapt, since cold temperatures can take your breath away.

1. Start by lying down or sitting comfortably.
2. Take 30 to 40 deep breaths. Inhale through your nose or mouth and exhale passively through your mouth. Fill your belly and your chest.
3. Hold your breath after the last inhale. After the last exhale, take 1 deep final inhalation, let the air out, and hold your breath until you feel you must breathe again.
4. When you must breathe again, take a deep breath and hold it for 15 seconds.
5. Repeat three to four times before your cold plunge or just as a simple, enlivening breath practice.

Cold Therapy

Cold therapy not only activates your metabolism but also stimulates dopamine, the focus, attention, and reward neurotransmitter. Practice cold therapy daily for 1 to 4 minutes. Here are some options.

1. Do the Wim Hof breath practice just described before your cold therapy.
2. Take a 1- to 2-minute cold shower every morning.
3. Fill up your bathtub with cold water and immerse yourself for 1 to 4 minutes.
4. For a little extra coldness, add ice to your bathtub.
5. Get a temperature-regulated cold plunge (which looks like a bathtub). See youngforever.com/resources on the best cold plunges.

Heat Therapy

The benefits of raising your body temperature are well established for well-being, mood, cardiovascular health, and longevity. Heat stress is an easy hack to feel better and live longer.

1. Take a hot bath regularly (three to four times a week). Try adding 500 grams of Epsom salts and 10 drops of lavender oil to help with sleep, muscle recovery, and lowering cortisol.

2. Get a home sauna. There are now many options, including a sauna blanket, small portable solo infrared sauna, or larger saunas. You can also get a steam shower easily installed in most home showers. This may be one of the best investments for your health. Or check out your local YMCA or gym to see if they have saunas. Ideally take a sauna four to five times a week for 30 minutes.

3. Hot yoga and vigorous exercise are other ways to boost your body temperature.

Phytohormesis: Leveraging Mother Nature for Longevity

Eating stressed-out plants makes you healthier and live longer. Our modern plants are too coddled, supported with fertilizer, herbicides, and pesticides and bred for higher yields and more starch, which has had horrible side effects. We have bred out most of the healing phytochemicals from our diet; the protein content and vitamins and minerals are lower, too. Try to incorporate wild and weird foods into your diet, such as wild greens, wild mushrooms, seaweed, dandelion greens, and heirloom varieties of vegetables. The next best phytochemical storehouses are regeneratively grown crops, then organic foods. Look for heirloom varieties. Shop at farmers' markets. Prioritize certain well-studied foods that activate all the longevity switches, including:

- Resveratrol, from red grapes
- Allicin, from garlic
- Capsaicin, from peppers

- Sulforaphane, from the broccoli family
- Curcumin, from turmeric
- Anthocyanins, from berries and black rice
- Quercetin and flavonoids, from Himalayan Tartary buckwheat, onions, and apples
- Epigallocatechin gallate (EGCG), from green tea
- Oleuropein, from extra virgin olive oil
- Phenolic acids, from mushrooms, including shiitake, maitake, and lion's mane

Try to incorporate the highest quality of these powerful phytohormetic plant compounds in your diet daily. Have green tea in the morning. Broccoli with garlic and onions. Himalayan Tartary buckwheat pancakes with apples. Dark green salads with extra virgin olive oil. Roasted mushrooms. And enjoy homemade curries with turmeric.

ADVANCED HORMESIS THERAPIES

Some promising hormesis treatments are a little harder to find or use but worth the effort if you have the time and money. These need not be done every day but can be used on a monthly or weekly basis.

Hyperbaric Oxygen Therapy: Oxygen under Pressure

The data on periodic use of hyperbaric oxygen chambers is exciting. Many cities have centers that offer "off-label" treatments. They can be expensive, but doing a 30- to 60-session course once a year can be a great addition to an advanced longevity regimen. Home hyperbaric oxygen units are also available, and though they can't reach the same level of pressure, they can still have great health and longevity benefits.

Hypoxia: Climbing Mount Everest

Unless you live at a higher altitude in a place like Colorado or Wyoming, you might find it hard to experience low-oxygen states, which are powerful at cleaning up old mitochondria and boosting cellular cleanup. However, there are some home devices, including the Cellgym, that can simulate a climb of Mount Everest. There are also respirator low-oxygen masks that limit the flow of oxygen; they can be used periodically during the day or during exercise to simulate low-oxygen states. They are often used by athletes for training. See youngforever book.com/resources for the best hypoxia masks. If you have any heart or lung disease, consult your doctor before trying this therapy.

Ozone Therapy

Ozone therapy sounds like a strange treatment, but as you learned in Chapter 10, it can be a powerful rejuvenating method to improve overall health. More and more practitioners are offering it, and home units are available that are safe for anyone to use (see youngforeverbook .com/resources).

Here are the typical options for ozone therapy.

1. **Home ozone generator,** which can be used for rectal or vaginal insufflation. You can do from 200 to 1,000 cc a day. This is delivered by filling a small bag with ozone connected to a rectal tube and slowly squeezed in over 10 to 15 minutes and held as long as you can, then released into the toilet. This can be done safely at home. See youngforeverbook.com/resources for affordable home ozone units.

2. **MAH or major autohemotherapy.** This technique removes your blood via gravity into a glass bottle, which is then infused with an ozone and oxygen mixture and then reinfused into the body. This and the rest of the ozone treatments that follow must be performed by a physician.

3. **Multipass ozone therapy or hyperbaric ozone therapy.** This technique removes blood via vacuum assist, then infuses it with ozone and oxygen. It is then returned to the body under pressure. Each cycle is equivalent to one MAH treatment, which usually takes

an hour. Using the hyperbaric ozone treatment, you can receive ten or more infusions or passes in less than an hour.

4. **Ozone dialysis.** This is a more advanced technique that removes your blood, runs it through a dialysis filter to clean it and ozonate it, and then reinfuses it.

Red-Light Therapy

More research is emerging that proves the benefits of red-light exposure for healing, pain relief, muscle recovery, improved lymphatic flow, immune function, collagen production, skin health, and mitochondrial health and cellular energy. Many home devices exist that can be used daily or whenever is convenient. See youngforeverbook .com/resources for the best devices.

We have covered all the foundational practices for extending both your health span and your life span: the Young Forever Longevity Diet, the right supplements, and the best lifestyle practices. Now we dive into how to personalize your approach to health and longevity by addressing your underlying unique imbalances in the seven core biological systems.

Chapter 17

The Young Forever Plan to Optimize Your Seven Core Biological Systems

> *Studying the interaction and interplay of many levels of biological information, systems biology will enable us to not only cure complex disease but to predict an individual's health and life span by preventive and personalized medicine made possible by the application of systems biology—representing a shift in the practice of medicine that will reach into many corners of our lives.*
>
> —Dr Leroy Hood, PhD, recipient of Lasker Award, Kyoto Prize, and Lemelson-MIT Prize; founder, Institute for Systems Biology

The Young Forever Program will help correct most of the imbalances in your seven core biological systems, but some people need more help to address deeper health issues. In Chapter 6 we reviewed how imbalances in our core biological networks are at the root of the hallmarks of aging. How do we correct those imbalances? With specific diet, lifestyle, supplement, drug, and hormesis therapies to optimize our biological networks.

Here's how to use this section of the book to personalize your health and longevity plan:

1. Take the quizzes in Chapter 13 to learn which of your core biological systems are out of balance. If your score is between 10 and 50 percent,

then you should focus on addressing that system by following the appropriate recommendations in this chapter. If your score is over 50 percent, you can apply the principles in this chapter, but if you are still not under 50 percent after implementing the strategies here, then find a good functional medicine doctor to help you address the remaining imbalances.

2. Get the Young Forever Function Health Panel (not available in the UK) as a baseline road map of testing.

3. Consider the additional tests outlined in Chapter 13 to diagnose imbalances in the systems where you scored over 50 percent. You will need to get most of these from a functional medicine doctor.

4. Implement the diet, lifestyle, and supplement recommendations that support the healing of your out-of-balance systems.

5. Start with Core System 1 (the gut) and Core System 2 (the immune system). These often help correct imbalances in all the other systems.

6. If you are still not feeling well or can't get your score below 10 percent, then it is important to follow up with a functional medicine practitioner (consult the website of the Institute for Functional Medicine, ifm.org).

The rest of this chapter will help you to heal the imbalances in your seven core biological systems. These can mostly be implemented on your own, but some people may need the help of a functional medicine doctor to be fully healed.

CORE SYSTEM 1: MICROBIOME AND GUT OPTIMIZATION

Healing the gut, tending our inner garden, can be the road back to health for so many people. It is essential for healthy aging and longevity. In fact, healing the gut is where I start with most of my patients.

How do we heal the gut? Here are the basic steps. I like to call it the weeding, seeding, and feeding program. Weed out the bad stuff, seed with probiotics, and feed the good bugs to heal the gut lining to repair a leaky gut.

1. **Remove potential allergens and inflammatory foods.** This is usually called an elimination diet. The top culprits are gluten, dairy, sugar, and alcohol. Grains and beans are next for many. Food additives, especially emulsifiers and thickeners, sugar alcohols, and artificial sweeteners are the worst.

2. **Stop gut-busting drugs,** including NSAIDs like ibuprofen or aspirin, antibiotics, steroids, and acid blockers. These may be needed from time to time for short-term symptom relief, but should not be taken long-term.

3. **Test for and treat parasites and overgrowth of bad bacteria and yeast.** See Chapter 13.

4. **Replenish digestive enzymes** with digestive enzyme tablets or capsules.

5. **Take prebiotic supplements and eat prebiotic foods,** including plantains, artichokes, asparagus, seaweed, jicama, dandelion greens, onions, and radicchio.

6. **Support the microbiome with probiotics.** There are many important probiotics that can help support different aspects of gut health and disease treatment. See youngforeverbook.com/resources for probiotic options. You can also increase probiotic foods such as miso, natto, tempeh, kimchi, sauerkraut, yogurt, and pickles.

7. **Increase intake of polyphenols** that support the microbiome: pomegranate, cranberry, green tea, curcumin, olive oil, and prickly pear—in fact, any colorful plant food.

8. **Consider using bovine immunoglobulins** (like colostrum) to support gut healing. There are dairy-free versions as well.

9. **Try Gut Food,** a product I created that contains highly researched probiotics, prebiotics, and polyphenols designed to provide long-term support for a healthy gut microbiome (gutfood.com).

10. **Fecal matter transplants (FMT)** may soon be routine for the treatment of many diseases and for supporting a healthy gut microbiome as we age, though much research is still needed to make this safe and effective.

CORE SYSTEM 2: IMMUNE AND INFLAMMATORY OPTIMIZATION

Inflammaging is both one of the hallmarks of aging and a root cause of many other hallmarks. The most powerful way to address the root causes of inflammation is to follow the Young Forever Program: heal the gut, minimize food allergens or sensitivities, reduce or eliminate environmental toxins, address latent infections, and learn to restore balance and reduce stress in your life.

In addition, certain therapies can be effective in addressing chronic inflammation and autoimmunity. Here are the main tools we use in functional medicine to address the root causes and restore optimal immune function.

1. **Eat an anti-inflammatory elimination diet.** The most powerful way to dramatically lower inflammation is to eliminate the most common inflammatory foods. I have written extensively about this and designed a clinically effective short-term diet to address inflammation. It is laid out in my book *The Blood Sugar Solution 10-Day Detox Diet* and eliminates sugar, starch, processed foods, gluten, dairy, grains, beans, coffee, and alcohol. In ten days, you can see remarkable results. We have seen an average 70 percent reduction in symptoms in all diseases in just ten days. Ideally the diet is continued for three months, or indefinitely if you find it works to relieve your symptoms and diseases.

2. **The autoimmune paleo diet** also eliminates nuts, seeds, eggs, and nightshades (tomatoes, peppers, potatoes, aubergines) and may be helpful for autoimmune disease, though the less restrictive 10-Day Detox Diet is effective for most people.

3. **Treat infections.** Most of us live with a host of viruses, bacteria, and parasites that our immune system manages. The balance can tip when our immune systems are suppressed. Think of a cold sore from a herpesvirus. The virus is latent but manifests under stress. The most common cause of chronic inflammation is either diagnosed or undiagnosed tick-borne infections such as Lyme disease. These may need to be treated with prescription and/or herbal antimicrobials.

However, other therapies such as ozone, hyperbaric oxygen, and hyperthermia (see later in this list) are often as or more effective in treating resistant infections than traditional antimicrobial therapy.

4. **Treat mold toxicity.** Undiagnosed mold exposure and toxicity are extremely common and treatable with the help of a functional medicine doctor experienced in mold toxicity.

5. **Use senolytics.** Zombie cells produce an inflammatory cascade that hastens disease and aging. Plant compounds such as quercetin, fisetin, curcumin, and newer drugs in development target and kill the zombie cells.

6. **Try peptides.** Peptides can also support immune function; they help address infections as well as support many aspects of healthy aging (see Chapter 11).

7. **Ozone therapy** is one of the most powerful germicidal and anti-inflammatory therapies available (see Chapter 16). It can be helpful in treating chronic infections, autoimmune disease, and inflammaging.[1]

8. **Hyperbaric oxygen therapy (HBOT)** is another effective strategy for helping to treat chronic infections (most bugs do not like oxygen). It has been shown to be one of the most powerful senolytics therapies, killing zombie cells.

9. **Hyperthermia,** a medical procedure used in Europe and Latin America but not yet available in the United States, can be very effective in treating chronic infections including tick-borne infections.[2] Our body naturally produces fever to kills infectious agents. Heating the body to high temperatures (up to 107°F/41°C) and using antimicrobials at the same time can be effective in treatment-resistant infections. It has also been used as a cancer treatment.[3]

10. **Consider exosomes.** Exosomes are little vesicles or packets of molecules produced by cells, including stem cells, that have shown promise in treating autoimmunity, infection, cancer, inflammation, and aging.[4] More science is needed, but exosomes will likely be a key therapeutic agent in medicine for a host of diseases and perhaps even aging itself. I have used them with significant benefit in healing of my back injuries and recovery from COVID-19. See Chapter 11.

CORE SYSTEM 3: MITOCHONDRIA AND ENERGY OPTIMIZATION

By now you know that our modern sugar- and starch-laden, processed diet is deadly for our mitochondria and turns off the longevity switches. Being sedentary and not strength training is guaranteed to accelerate aging because of its harmful effects on your mitochondria. Revive your mitochondria, increase their number and function, and boost your energy and longevity with these options:

1. **Follow the Young Forever Longevity Diet** (see Chapter 14), which is low in starch and sugar and high in good fats and phytochemicals.

2. **Eliminate or reduce environmental toxins** (see "Core System 4: Detoxification Optimization" later in this chapter).

3. **Practice hormesis daily** (see Chapter 16). Time-restricted eating, intermittent fasting, ketogenic diets, phytohormesis foods and spices, strength and HIIT training, cold and hot therapies, hyperbaric oxygen, hypoxia practices, breath work, and ozone therapy all support mitochondria. Include as many of these practices as you can.

4. **Take the Young Forever Supplements** (see Chapter 15).

5. **Consider additional mitochondria therapy,** depending on your health status and testing (with a functional medicine doctor): coenzyme Q10 or PQQ, alpha-lipoic acid, and acetyl-L-carnitine. See Advanced Longevity Support Supplements (page 236 in Chapter 15).

6. **Also consider NMN, pterostilbene, and urolithin A (Mitopure)** (see Chapter 15).

7. **Use red-light therapy** (see Chapter 10) to boost energy production in the mitochondria.

8. **Consider peptide therapy,** such as SS 31, humanin, and MOTs-C. Peptides are little proteins that modulate most aspects of our biology, including our mitochondria. They are now available mostly as subcutaneous injections (see Chapter 11).

9. **Consider calorie-restriction-mimicking therapies** such as rapamycin and metformin (I do not routinely prescribe these and think we need more data on humans before we recommend their use in medical practice, but they may turn out to produce the same benefits on the mitochondria as calorie restriction, without eating less. See Chapter 15).

CORE SYSTEM 4: DETOXIFICATION OPTIMIZATION

Sadly, our world is awash in a sea of toxins, from the food we eat to the water we drink, the air we breathe, and the home care and personal care products we use. Here are some simple strategies to lower your toxic exposures and support your detox systems to eliminate stored toxins.

1. **Reduce toxic exposures.**
   * Do your best to eat organic food or regeneratively raised food.
   * Use the Pesticide Action Network's Dirty Dozen and alternatives as a guide to which fruits and vegetables are the most or least contaminated (pan-uk.org).
   * Filter your water, ideally with a reverse osmosis filter, and get an air filter for your home. The ones I recommend can be found at drhyman.com/filter.
   * Eliminate high-mercury fish. Use the Good Fish Guide produced by the Marine Conservation Society (mcsuk.org).
   * Eliminate toxic household cleaning products and personal care products. Use the Pesticide Action Network's guides (pan-uk.org).
2. **Enhance your body's detoxification systems.**
   * Drink 8 to 10 glasses of filtered water a day.
   * Have one to two bowel movements a day. If you are constipated, try magnesium citrate, buffered vitamin C, probiotics,

and fiber such as flaxseeds and chia seeds. If you are still struggling, see a functional medicine doctor for further evaluation.
- Sweat daily with exercise, saunas, steam, or hot baths.

3. **Upregulate your detoxification pathways.**
    - *Consume detoxifying foods daily,* including 100 to 200 grams of cruciferous vegetables, garlic, onions, artichokes, watercress, beets, avocados, lemons, green tea, ginger, rosemary, and turmeric (see Chapter 7 for more on food and detoxification).
    - *Take supplements that support detoxification.* The liver has many pathways for detoxification that require vitamins, minerals, and amino acids. The B vitamins, especially folate, B_{12}, and B_6; selenium; zinc; and magnesium are the most essential.
    - *Support glutathione,* which is the most important detoxifying molecule made by your body, from the amino acids glycine, cysteine, and glutamine. Goat or regeneratively raised A2 cows' whey, cruciferous vegetables, garlic, and onions boost glutathione production. Supplements and herbs that are effective in boosting detoxification include n-acetylcysteine, alpha-lipoic acid, milk thistle, and curcumin.
    - Intravenous support with glutathione can be a way to periodically support detoxification.

4. **Treat your heavy metal burden.** If you have a high risk of metals from fish intake or amalgam fillings or live in a polluted environment, a heavy metal chelation challenge test is important to assess your total-body burden. It is often necessary to use chelators such as DMSA or EDTA to remove metals. Work with a functional medicine doctor to assess and treat high levels of toxic burden.

5. **Address mold toxicity.** If you suspect that you have had mold exposure, work with a functional medicine doctor to test for it and treat it with antifungals and binders. It is also important to identify and remove the source of mold, which may require a mold expert to evaluate your home, followed by remediation.

CORE SYSTEM 5: OPTIMIZING COMMUNICATION, HORMONE BALANCE, AND METABOLIC HEALTH

Optimize Glucose and Insulin Metabolism

The single most important thing you can do to prevent and reverse disease and extend your healthy life span is to keep your insulin low and your blood sugar in balance. How can we best do this?

1. **Consume** a low-refined-carbohydrate, higher-fat, high-fiber, phytonutrient-rich diet.

2. **Consider my book** *The Blood Sugar Solution 10-Day Detox Diet* to address sugar addiction and reset your biology (see youngforeverbook .com/resources).

3. **Consider a ketogenic diet** if you have type 2 diabetes, until your diabetes is reversed.

4. **Exercise.** Build muscle and optimize your VO$_2$ max.

5. **Take the Core Supplement Plan** (see Chapter 15), which includes magnesium, chromium, biotin, vitamin D, and omega-3 fats, which all support optimal glucose control.

6. **Add the Advanced Longevity Support Supplements** (see Chapter 15), which benefit insulin signaling, the sirtuin pathway, and AMPK to improve insulin sensitivity and glucose control.

7. **Add alpha-lipoic acid,** 600 mg twice a day, and berberine, 1 g a day (such as CM Core by Ortho Molecular Products).

8. **Address causes of inflammation,** including dysbiosis and environmental toxins.

9. **Research a potential prescription for metformin,** 500 mg before lunch and dinner. If your blood sugar is ideal, though, metformin's longevity benefits are as yet unproven. Consult with your doctor.

10. **Use a continuous glucose monitor** to track your response to food. Try Levels Health to track your blood sugar and progress (levelshealth.com/hyman). A similar system is available from FreeStyle Libre (freestylelibre.co.uk).

Hormone Optimization Therapy

Modern life is mostly a disaster for our hormones, especially our sex hormones, thyroid, and adrenal or stress hormones. Following the Young Forever Program will help to optimize most hormones. However, some of us may need extra support as we age.

Bioidentical Hormone Optimization

Both women and men experience hormonal changes with chronological age: menopause and andropause. Sugar and starch, alcohol, caffeine, sedentary lifestyle, stress, and environmental toxins all manifest as hormonal imbalances in men and women. Women who follow a healthy lifestyle often suffer minimal symptoms of menopause, such as hot flushes, mood changes, sleep problems, low libido, and vaginal dryness. Hormonal imbalances in men occur from lower testosterone driven by insulin resistance, stress, and lack of exercise, especially strength training. Symptoms include loss of muscle, fatigue, low motivation, low sex drive, and erectile dysfunction.

The first order of business is to address the causes. Then, if symptoms persist, you might consider hormone therapy. Here are the basic rules for hormone therapy:

1. **Use only bioidentical hormones** (the same forms made by your body).
2. **Use the lowest dose possible.**
3. **Use for as short a time as possible.**
4. **Use topically or by injection.**
5. **Ideally, work with a functional medicine doctor** experienced in hormone therapy.

Women's Hormone Optimization

The science of hormone therapy for women has gone through considerable ups and downs. Common hormone replacement therapies are

Premarin (horse estrogen) and Provera (a synthetic progesterone). Premarin has significant side effects, including higher risk of heart attack, inflammation, stroke, and female cancers. Provera causes weight gain, facial hair, and depression. However, bioidentical hormone therapy may not have the same risks. These are human or bioidentical hormones, which are usually much better tolerated with fewer side effects and risks.

My general approach is to use short-term therapy for symptoms of menopause that subside after a few years. Most eighty-year-old women don't have hot flushes! Low-dose longer-term therapy for ongoing symptoms can be safely done with careful monitoring of breast, uterine, cervical, and ovarian health. It is important to see a gynecologist for breast exams, mammograms, Pap tests, and intravaginal ultrasound before starting any therapy, as well as for a yearly assessment. If treatment is needed, these are the best options:

1. **Topical bioidentical estradiol and progesterone** (creams, gels, drops, patches).
2. **Vaginal estradiol** (creams or tablets such as Vagifem) to address vaginal dryness.
3. **Low-dose testosterone** for low libido, which can be added to compounded creams, gels, or drops.
4. **Clitoral testosterone drops,** 5mg/mL, 2 drops each night— from a compounding pharmacy. This can be very effective for low libido when taken consistently.
5. **Peptide therapy.** PT 141, also known as bremelanotide, is effective for enhancing libido and sexual function in both men and women.

Men's Hormone Optimization

Testosterone can be used as an interim therapy to help obese men with very low testosterone (<500 ng/dL) build muscle, lose weight, and optimize the benefits of exercise. Older men with low libido and erectile function or sarcopenia may also benefit from testosterone therapy. The best ways to boost testosterone naturally are to eat good fats, including saturated fat (all sex hormones are made from cholesterol); engage in stress-reduction practices, such as meditation; and do strength training. Risks of testosterone therapy include elevation of cholesterol, thickening of the blood, and stimulation of latent prostate cancer. Careful evaluation and review by your physician are important to make sure it is safe for you. If treatment is needed, these are the best options:

1. **Intramuscular injections of testosterone,** usually 80 to 100 mg a week to achieve a testosterone level between 500 and 1,000 ng/dL.

2. **Topical testosterone gels or creams** such as AndroGel or Testostim.

3. **Implantable testosterone pellets.**

4. **Peptide therapy.** PT 141, also known as bremelanotide, is effective for enhancing libido and erections in men and can be used in combination with drugs such as Viagra or Cialis.

Thyroid Hormone Replacement

One in five women and one in ten men suffer low thyroid function. This can result in increased risk of heart disease, memory loss, depression, fatigue, muscle loss, low libido, hair loss, constipation, and dry skin and hair. Gluten and environmental toxins are common causes of thyroid dysfunction. Many who are diagnosed are not adequately treated because most physicians use the inactive form of thyroid, T4 or levothyroxine, which doesn't work for everyone. It is important to do the correct tests (see Chapter 13) because most physicians just check TSH, which will miss many cases of thyroid dysfunction. I have written an ebook, *The Ultra Thyroid Solution,* that explains in detail how to assess thyroid dysfunction, identify the causes, and optimally treat the thyroid. You can learn more at drhyman.com/ty-thyroid. If you need thyroid replacement, here's what I recommend.

1. Use bioidentical thyroid replacement.
2. Use a combination of levothyroxine (T4), the inactive hormone, and liothyronine (T3), the active hormone. Dosing must be personalized and adjusted with your doctor.
3. Ideally use desiccated porcine thyroid, which contains all the compounds in the appropriate balance to support optimal thyroid function, including T4, T3, and T2. Brands include Armour Thyroid and Nature-Throid.

Adrenal Support

As we age, we become less stress resilient. Sugar, starch, alcohol, stress, lack of adequate sleep, caffeine, and late eating all burden our adrenal glands. Our adrenal glands help us respond to stress by releasing cortisol and adrenaline. However, chronic long-term stress at first overstimulates the adrenals, causing high cortisol and adrenaline. Over time your adrenals can't keep up and become "fatigued"; they can't produce cortisol in response to stress. That results in adrenal burnout. The key to restoring adrenal function is to focus on living a healthy lifestyle. Nutritional and herbal supplements can be helpful and, rarely, adrenal hormone support may be needed. Here are the key strategies to avoid adrenal burnout and optimize your adrenal function.

1. **Wake and sleep at the same time daily.**
2. **Get exposure to morning sunlight** for 20 minutes a day.
3. **Eliminate blue-light exposure at night** with blue-blocker glasses, and use red-light bulbs.
4. **Exercise,** but don't overexercise (not usually a problem unless you run marathons).
5. **Avoid sugar and starch,** which cause elevated cortisol and adrenaline.
6. **Practice a stress-reduction strategy daily,** such as breath work, yoga, meditation, massage, or a hot bath or sauna.

7. **Take the Young Forever Core Supplement Plan.** Vitamin C, B vitamins, and magnesium all help adrenal function.

8. **Consider herbal support,** including adaptogenic mushrooms like cordyceps and reishi, and herbs like rhodiola, Siberian ginseng, ginseng, and ashwagandha.

9. **Low doses of DHEA** (an adrenal hormone) can improve energy and overall well-being. Women can start at 10 mg and go up to 50 mg and men can start at 25 mg and go up to 50 mg. This can have some androgenic effects—for women it can increase facial hair and for men it can cause hair loss.

Growth Hormone

Human growth hormone (HGH) is essential for physical growth and appropriate body mass. It is secreted in the anterior pituitary and found in your brain, and it controls growth in children and helps maintain stature in adults. HGH is important for stimulating the breakdown of triglycerides and keeps excess fat from being stored, helps build protein and muscles, and plays a role in helping maintain normal blood sugar levels. HGH declines as we age, which results in a decrease in muscle mass, libido, and energy and an increase in fat storage. Certain lifestyle interventions, such as balancing blood sugar, exercising, and practicing intermittent fasting, can help to improve production.

For many years antiaging physicians promoted the use of growth hormone for longevity and performance. While growth hormone declines as we chronologically age, it can be naturally increased by supporting your adrenal function (see previously in this chapter), optimizing sleep, weight training, and even peptide therapy (see Chapter 11). Giving growth hormone directly can increase the risk of diabetes and may increase cancer risk. Given all the other options for extending your health span and life span, growth hormone replacement is not on my recommended list of safe and effective therapies.

CORE SYSTEM 6: TRANSPORT OPTIMIZATION

Keeping things flowing in the body is essential for cellular communication and detoxification. Keeping your blood and lymph systems in good working order is a cornerstone of good health and optimal aging.

1. **Eat the Young Forever Longevity Diet,** which includes many foods that help improve blood vessel and lymph health.

2. **Move.** Any type of exercise supports the health of your circulatory system and lymphatic circulation.

3. **Start a regular yoga practice.** Combining deep breathing and stretching is one of the most powerful detoxifying practices and supports your lymph flow and stimulation of your intestines, liver, and kidneys. Hot yoga gives the added benefit of sweating. Also, consider a daily Wim Hof breathing practice, outlined in Chapter 16. This moves (or exercises) the diaphragm, the main muscle that brings lymph flow back into your heart.

4. **Use sauna therapy or take hot baths regularly.** This increases circulation and helps reset your nervous system and boosts your overall health and longevity.

5. **Follow heat therapy with a cold plunge.** The cold helps to boost lymph circulation.[5]

6. **Get massage regularly if you can,** especially lymphatic massage. This helps flush out muscles and supports lymph flow.

7. **Try muscle-recovery devices** that passively increase lymph flow using pneumatic compression of lower extremities, such as Hyperice (hyperice.com).

CORE SYSTEM 7: STRUCTURAL OPTIMIZATION

As we age, our bodies get banged up, leading to chronic pain and limitations in activity and motion. The more pain we have, the less we move. The less we move, the faster we age. Advances in therapies to improve function and relieve pain have revolutionized the way we can and will care for our musculoskeletal system. This is often referred to as *regenerative medicine*.

I have had to rehabilitate myself from decades of chronic pain. With a combination of body work, yoga, the TB12 Sports physical therapy and training program, and seeing a regenerative medicine doctor, I have become stronger, fitter, and more pain-free than I have been in 30 years. Here are the top ways to keep your meat suit in good working order and to repair and heal it when you need help.

1. **Engage in regular exercise,** including aerobic conditioning, strength training, and flexibility. I am a huge advocate of the TB12 Sports program developed by Tom Brady to keep him active, pain-free, strong, and winning into his midforties. The program uses resistance bands and specially designed workouts and vibrating foam rollers to increase muscle pliability and to reduce injury and pain. They have an app or you can work with one of their body coaches on Zoom (tb12sports.com). The TB12 Sports band-training program is my staple for strength training.

2. **Yoga** is a powerful way to help the body relieve pain and decrease stress and can be done at any age.

3. **Supplements** can help build muscle, repair tissues and joints, and reduce inflammation. Try omega fats such as Dutch Harbor Omega with high levels of inflammation-suppressing resolvins; Zyflamend by New Chapter, an anti-inflammatory herbal mixture; collagen peptides; bone broth; and glucosamine.

4. **Peptide therapy** with BPC-157, thymosin beta-4 fragments, and GHK can help reduce pain and repair injured tissues and joints. See youngforeverbook.com/resources for how to purchase and use peptides.

5. **Work with a physical therapist and body coach** if you have chronic issues. After my last back surgery I used the TB12 Sports body coaches, who are trained in a special form of physical therapy that helps get to the root of the problems and heal chronic injuries.

6. **Try Prolozone therapy** if you have chronic joint pain or arthritis. Small amounts of ozone and oxygen are injected into joints

or tissues, which promotes healing and regeneration of tissues.[6] It is more effective than most current joint treatments. It has helped my patients headed for knee surgery walk pain-free again and cured my frozen shoulder in 5 minutes.

7. **Try massage devices** like the Theragun or Hypervolt.

8. **Work with a regenerative medicine doctor.** Consider a combination of regenerative therapies, including peptides, exosomes, stem cells, placental matrix, and hydro-dissection of fascia, nerves, and muscles to promote healing and regeneration (see Chapter 11). For me, regenerative medicine has been nothing short of miraculous. These therapies are not widely available yet but are becoming more and more available through regenerative medicine clinics around the United States. They will prove to be essential in the field of orthopedics and pain management.

OPTIMIZING NUTRITIONAL STATUS

If you scored over 10 percent in any of the nutrient-deficiency quizzes, you may need extra nutritional support. The Core Supplement Plan covers most of the bases, with B vitamins, vitamin D, magnesium, omega-3 fats, and zinc. However, if you have a significant issue with methylation, you may need higher doses of specialized forms of vitamin B_{12}, B_6, and folate.

1. **Take the Core Supplement Plan.**

2. **Add Homocysteine Supreme** by Designs for Health if you have a high homocysteine level on your Young Forever Function Health Panel or a score of more than 50 percent on the methylation quiz.

OPTIMIZING MIND-BODY-SPIRIT HEALING

Perhaps the hardest aspect of healing is healing our mind, our heart, and our spirit. This has been the work of shamans and spiritual healers for thousands of years. Several new and important revolutionary approaches exist. Some you may be familiar with, and others may sound strange, but emerging research in the last decade has brought game-changing disruptive approaches to the forefront.

Here are a few avenues to explore to heal deep-seated childhood conditioning, trauma, anxiety, and depression, and even to help you find your own meaning and purpose.

1. **Get support.** Try therapy, counseling, or coaching. I have found that a life coach can be extremely helpful in examining your life, behaviors, and patterns and in holding you accountable to the changes you want to make in your life. I have used the Handel Group for my own personal coaching, and it has profoundly changed how I feel and live. They have an online self-guided program called Inner.U that includes ways to get support from others. Learn more at handelgroup.com.

2. **Try dynamic neural retraining,** an online program that can help heal the chronic stress and trauma we all experience that keeps us in a state of fight, flight, or freeze. It targets brain function to regulate a maladapted stress response and teaches you how to rewire the limbic system (emotional center of the brain) and change the structure and function of your brain. This allows your body to move from a state of survival to a state of growth and repair, where true healing can take place (see Dynamic Neural Retraining System, retrainingthebrain.com).

3. **Try ketamine therapy** for anxiety, depression, and post-traumatic stress disorder (PTSD). Ketamine is an anesthetic drug that is now approved for treatment of resistant depression.[7] The FDA approved a nasal spray called Spravato. It is a dissociative drug that allows you to see things from a different perspective. It also has direct effects on healing brain function and structure, increasing neuroplasticity. Ketamine clinics are now legal and can be found in nearly every major city.

4. **Try a stellate ganglion block** for anxiety, trauma, and PTSD.[8] Since the 1940s, stellate ganglion blocks have been performed to treat pain conditions driven by the sympathetic or stress response in the nervous system. The procedure involves injecting local anesthetic

in and around the stellate ganglion, a bundle of nerves in the sympathetic nervous system (located at the base of the neck) to temporarily block its function. Hospitals and clinics that perform this treatment can be found all over the country. You can learn more at the website for Stella (stellacenter.com). The procedure usually involves one or two sessions and can have long-lasting effects.

5. **Explore emerging psychedelic treatments** for mental, emotional, and spiritual health.[9] Millions of dollars are now flooding into research, and billion-dollar companies have emerged to take advantage of this revolution in mental health care. The Multidisciplinary Association for Psychedelic Studies is advancing the research on the use of psilocybin (magic mushrooms), LSD, MDMA (known as a party drug called Ecstasy), and ayahuasca as treatments for depression, anxiety, and PSTD as well as palliative-care treatments. Learn more about this research at their website, maps.org. Psychedelics have a long history of use in ancient cultures—peyote by Native Americans, bufo or 5 MeO-DMT from the Sonoran Desert toad, ayahuasca and San Pedro cactus (mescalin) by the shamans of South America, and iboga from the healers of Gabon in West Africa. Watch the Netflix series *How to Change Your Mind,* based on the book by Michael Pollan, or read the book, to learn more. There are clinics in Mexico and Central America that offer these treatments now.

6. **Explore ibogaine therapy for PTSD and addiction.** One psychedelic seems to have very unusual and powerful effects in treating addiction in addition to PTSD and depression. Ibogaine is a psychoactive alkaloid that has been used historically in healing ceremonies and initiations by members of the Bwiti religion in various parts of West Africa. People with problematic substance use have found that larger doses of ibogaine can significantly reduce withdrawal from opiates and temporarily eliminate substance-related cravings.[10] Research is underway that may revolutionize the treatment of addiction. Ibogaine can have serious cardiac side effects and is always delivered in a medically supervised environment. Derivative compounds like noribogaine that may not have the same adverse side effects are under

development. There are clinics in Mexico and Central America that offer these treatments now.

Congratulations! You have made it through the science of aging and learned how to implement the foundational practices of the Young Forever Program. You have also learned how to personalize your program based on your laboratory results and quizzes. Start where you can; choose the things that inspire you. Habit change is not always easy. Organize your house, your kitchen, and your bedroom to make it easy to do the right things. Get support. Do it with a friend. Start a Young Forever group where you can help and encourage one another. We know that our social environment determines so much about our health, that our family and friends shape our health behaviors.

Think of the Young Forever Program as a road map for your journey to health and longevity. Heed the old Chinese proverb "A journey of a thousand miles begins with one step." Take the first step.

Next, I will share my own personal health and longevity practices, taking you through how I integrate the science of health and longevity into my own life.

Chapter 18

Dr Hyman's Young Forever Program: Putting It All Together

I arise in the morning torn between a desire to improve the world and
a desire to enjoy the world. This makes it hard to plan the day.
                                                    —E. B. WHITE

Many wonder how I have managed to stay strong, healthy, and youthful at sixty-three when many of my peers are winding down. I am helicopter skiing, dramatically improving my tennis game, building more muscle, and outperforming my thirty-year-old friends bike riding up a mountain and lifting heavier weights. My goal is not just to leave my biological age at forty-three but to continue to turn back the clock to twenty-five! Next, I share the weekly practices that are keeping me biologically younger as I grow chronologically older.

DR HYMAN'S LONGEVITY PROGRAM

Knowing all the possibilities to slow or reverse aging may be exciting or overwhelming. How do you possibly choose the best options for yourself? You have to choose what resonates with you, what you can incorporate in your life on a regular basis. You can't do everything at once, but over time you can explore different avenues to support and enhance your health and well-being and help you live a long, vibrant, active life. Here's my day-to-day longevity lifestyle.

Diet

- I follow the Pegan Diet, focused on high levels of phytochemicals, especially those known to support the longevity pathways and work on the hallmarks of aging.
- I drink my Healthy Aging Shake (page 230) daily within an hour of exercise to build muscle.

Exercise

- Four to six days of aerobic exercise with interval training, including road and mountain biking, tennis, hiking, and swimming, for an average of 30 to 60 minutes a session.
- Strength training using TB12 Sports resistance bands and the TB12 Sports workout app three to four times a week for 30 minutes.
- Hot yoga or vinyasa yoga twice a week and daily shorter yoga/stretch sessions.

Sleep

- 7 to 8 hours a night. I am usually asleep by 10 p.m. or 11 p.m. and wake by 6 a.m. or 7 a.m.
- Magnesium glycinate, 200 to 400 mg a night.
- Eyeshades and earplugs to create a light- and soundproof environment.
- Sleep and biomarker tracking with the Oura Ring and Eight Sleep system.

Stress Management

- 20 minutes of mantra meditation once or twice a day.
- Breath work ideally daily.
- I prioritize spending time in nature and the wilderness; it restores my nervous system and inspires me.

- I spend time with friends and family in play and adventure whenever I can (and I make it a priority).
- I get massages at least once a month (more if I can!).

Hormesis

- I practice time-restricted eating with a 14- to 16-hour window three to four times a week.
- I include the most potent phytohormesis plant compounds in my diet on a regular basis.
- When I have access to saunas and cold plunges, I do them daily. At home I have a steam shower and a big bathtub I fill with ice-cold water and do a few rounds of therapy daily—10 minutes in the steam, then 3 minutes in the cold bath. I spend 30 minutes three to four times a week in my sauna when home or do hot yoga when I am on the road.
- I use a red-light therapy device as often as I can when I am home, for 10 minutes a day.
- I use blue-blocker glasses at night.
- I use ozone therapy weekly as a tune-up when I am home or have access to it. Even monthly is a good hormetic reset.
- I have used hyperbaric oxygen therapy to reset my system once a year but not as a regular therapy (yet).
- I use the Cellgym machine for hypoxia training when I have access to one at a health or biohacking center, and I use a low-oxygen mask while working at my desk.

Basic Supplement Plan

- Vitamin D Supreme by Designs for Health (vitamin D_3, 5,000 IU a day with vitamin K_2, including MK-7 form)
- Dutch Harbor Omega (EPA/DHA, 1 to 2 g a day) or other brands of Alaskan cod liver oil
- Multi t/d by Pure Encapsulations, 2 a day (multivitamin and mineral)

- Homocysteine Supreme by Designs for Health, 2 a day (methylation support with B_6, B_{12}, and folate because my methylation genes need extra help)
- Magnesium glycinate by Pure Encapsulations, 400 mg a day
- Gut Food from Farmacy for gut support (gutfood.com)

Longevity Stack

- NMN, 1,000 mg a day
- Fisetin, 500 mg a day
- HTB Rejuvenate by Big Bold Health with quercetin and other flavonols, 2 twice a day
- Pterostilbene, 100 mg once or twice a day
- Curcumin with Bioprene, 500 mg a day
- Epigallocatechin gallate, 500 mg a day from green tea
- OncoPLEX by Xymogen (sulforaphane from broccoli seed extract), 30 mg twice a day
- Mitopure (urolithin A), 500 mg a day, 1 packet or 2 capsules a day

Sarcopenia Support

- Amino Acid Complex from Thorne Research, 1 scoop a day after workout
- Creatine, 5 grams daily in my Healthy Aging Shake (page 230)

ADVANCED LONGEVITY THERAPIES

I have explored many emerging therapies, using myself as guinea pig. I find them very helpful in improving my overall health and well-being and for addressing chronic injuries. I have had many health challenges, including autoimmune disease, mold toxicity, mercury poisoning, Lyme disease, and back injuries, and use these to uplevel my health. They are part of what is known as regenerative medicine. They all need more research to be ready for prime time. Following are the ones I have found most helpful. Those of you who are longevity pioneers and explorers may want to explore them, but do consult with your doctor before trying any of them. The cost of these therapies is very high today but will, in time, become more affordable and even covered by insurance. See Chapter 11.

Here are the advanced therapies I have tried as part of my overall health and longevity regimen. Remember, I have chosen to try these knowing the potential risks and that more research is needed. Each of us has a different appetite for exploration and budget. You can choose to explore all or none of these:

- Peptide therapy
- Exosomes
- Stem cells
- Natural killer cell infusions
- Transfer plasma exchange (TPE), a more palatable approach to cleaning the blood than parabiosis

Meaning, Purpose, and Mental Health

- I am blessed to have found meaningful work that helps serve others as a physician, author, and podcast host of *The Doctor's Farmacy*. I have a nonprofit, Food Fix Campaign (foodfix.org), that is actively working to create a healthier and more equitable food system for all by addressing the need to improve our food and agricultural policies.
- I have worked hard on my mental health and mindset, and I get support from my life coach and friends. Exploring spiritual traditions has been helpful for me.

Community and Connection

- Each week I gather on Zoom with six of my closest long-term male friends for a support group where we each are deeply known and seen and encouraged to grow and develop ourselves professionally and personally.
- I have been very deliberate about cultivating a wonderful community of friends and colleagues who know me and provide a deep sense of love and belonging.

Afterword

The Perils and Promise of Our Time

It was the best of times, it was the worst of times, it was the age of wisdom, it was the age of foolishness, it was the epoch of belief, it was the epoch of incredulity, it was the season of Light, it was the season of Darkness, it was the spring of hope, it was the winter of despair, we had everything before us, we had nothing before us, we were all going direct to Heaven, we were all going direct the other way.
— CHARLES DICKENS, *A TALE OF TWO CITIES*

We are at a remarkable time in human history. What was science fiction is now science fact—cars, planes, space travel, supercomputers in our pockets. What now seems like science fiction will soon become commonplace. It is hard for our linear human minds to comprehend what's coming next. We have seen the promise of longevity science and its potential to reprogram our biology back to its youthful state, advances that hold the potential of immortality, which mortals have longed for since the Holy Grail. Throughout most of our ancestral history, change has been slow and plodding. It is now exponential. And with that change we have seen miracles, like organ transplants and men on the moon.

But we have also seen massive destruction wrought through the unintended consequences of our forward progress and ingenuity. We have lost 60 percent of species to extinction due to human activity, created massive deserts, destroyed rain forests, depleted and poisoned our freshwater supplies, polluted our planet, and destabilized our climate, threatening the very survival of the human species. Just as we are on the verge of living as long as Methuselah, we are simultaneously facing our own extinction in the near future.

It is easy to be pessimistic about the state of the world today. The rise of autocracies, the decline of democracy, the growing economic and health inequities, the rapidly heating climate threatening to destabilize governments and populations, the polarization of our society, the rise of hate and discrimination, the erosion of human rights, the dramatic increase in global obesity and chronic disease, the destructive food system, the usurping of free will through the digital persuasion economy that controls our choices, beliefs, and behaviors through manipulative algorithms, are enough to make it hard to get out of bed in the morning. But at the same time as we face these big, hairy problems, we are also discovering how to solve our most audacious challenges through innovation, creativity, and the genius of the human mind and spirit.

It is not a foregone conclusion that we will survive, and many before, including Thomas Malthus and Paul Ehrlich in his book *The Population Bomb,* have portended an end to our species and predicted a future where population growth would outstrip the capacity of the Earth to sustain us. Those predictions have not come to be, because humans seem to always pull the proverbial rabbit out of the hat. We may do so this time or not, but as a doctor, I see the potential to heal both our bodies and our minds, to repair broken societies, and to heal a damaged planet.

Abraham Lincoln implored us to search for our better angels, to overcome moments in history fraught with danger, where our baser instincts and desires are sublimated to a more enlightened perspective focused on raising one another out of darkness. We are in that moment now.

The focus on longevity and life extension for its own sake might seem like a narcissistic pursuit of the wealthy or a distraction from the fear of death. But for me, the promise of healing, of relieving the needless suffering of billions of people from the ravages of disease, disability, and frailty, the promise of helping humans become the best versions of themselves by healing their bodies, by healing our individual and collective trauma, by reimagining society and ways of being that bring more joy, creativity, art, music, love, wonder, and magic into the world, is the only work that I am called to do. To unburden humanity from our own baser instincts through our ingenuity, creativity, science, and imagination. To reimagine how we can live in ways that are in harmony with one another and the Earth.

The revolution in medicine promises to transform everything we know about health, disease, and aging, relegating the common diseases of today, like heart disease, cancer, diabetes, and dementia, to the dustbin of history, just as we vanquished smallpox. Advances in technology will soon allow energy abundance without fossil fuels. Regenerative ways of growing our food and living are emerging at an exponential rate. Billions of dollars in investment and in philanthropy are directed at solving our most vexing problems. How it all turns out remains to be seen, but my belief is that if we start with our own healing, both our bodies and our minds, we will reclaim what our stressed-out, inflammatory society has taken from us, our cooperative nature, our ability to work together and to live in balance with one another and the Earth.

My hope is that the lessons learned in this book, the tools that can relieve suffering, end disease, and extend the time we can each be healthy and contribute to our families, communities, and society, will create a kinder, more compassionate world. Personally, my goal of living to 120 or 180 is born not from a hedonistic pursuit but from the fact that, finally, at the age of sixty-three, I feel I have the wisdom and the capacity to add so much more value to the world, to my family, and to my community, and to help solve some of our most challenging problems. There seems to be no other more important work for us today.

Mark Hyman
October 2022

Acknowledgments

Every book is a collective work. This book is possible only because of the heroic, tireless work of scientists over many decades asking the hard questions, exploring the mystery and potential of human life. It is to them that I owe much gratitude and thanks. My work is primarily as a translator and doctor, translating science buried in journals, work done in obscure laboratories, and insights from my decades of clinical care into simple, practical recommendations and tools to improve our lot as human beings. It has been the honor of my life to do this work.

I have learned from so many, including leading giants in the field of longevity, especially my friends David Sinclair and Valter Longo. Dan Buettner has been a remarkable friend and inspiration, making the secrets of the Blue Zones known to the world. He helped guide my journeys to Sardinia and Ikaria, where he connected me to Eleonora Catta and Paola Demurtas, who, through their travel company, There, took me on a deep journey into the heart of the Sardinian Blue Zone. And to Eleni Mazari from Ikaria, who introduced me to the old ways. I am grateful for the friendship and support of Tony Robbins and Peter Diamandis, who wrote *Life Force*. They hold the vision of a healed abundant future that keeps me inspired, and invited me to help them create that future.

And, as always, I have been supported by my extraordinary team: Dhru Purohit, my business partner and CEO of everything Hyman, who brings his heart, genius, and integrity to everything and everyone. Kaya Purohit, my head of content, who turns all my crazy ideas and content into digestible, actionable ideas and tools that help millions. A special thanks to Darci Gross, who helped me massage the manuscript, making the promise of the book accessible and easy to understand. Farrell Feighan, Lauren Feighan, Alex Gallegos, Ben

Tseitlin, Harshal Purohit-Patel, Ailsa Cowell, Gerry Doherty, Patrick Edwards, Melanie Haraldson, Kay Lemus, Courtney McNary, Ayelet Menashe, Jennifer Sanders, Susan Verity, Linda Cardillo, Harrison King, Taylor Groff, Hannah Ordos, Amber Cox, Carol Syversen, Dianna Towns, Loren Gould, Mara Floyd, and Mary Workman are the best team in the world.

Without Meredith Jones, most of my life would not be possible. She makes everything easy for me, makes sure I know what to do when, and frees up my mind so I can do the work I came to do. Thank you!

My patients over the last 30 years have trusted me with their health and taught me so much about the true meaning of being a doctor, and about how the human body truly works. Thank you. My teams at The UltraWellness Center and the Cleveland Clinic Center for Functional Medicine hold down the fort while I continue to learn and explore the future of science and medicine. Without Dr Jeffrey Bland, my mentor and friend, an unsung hero and the greatest visionary of twenty-first-century medicine, I would not be alive, and certainly would not have had the knowledge and skills to heal myself and so many.

My longtime agent, Richard Pine, and my editor, Tracy Behar at Little, Brown Spark, have supported me and welcomed my crazy ideas over the last 20 years. None of what I have been able to bring to the world would have happened without you and your trust in me. And as always, Andrea Vinley Converse helped me shape the manuscript into something that is accessible to all, and put up with my resistance to cut out words (that needed cutting).

To my community of friends and my family, who keep me grounded and full of love and support, I couldn't do life without any of you. My daughter, Rachel, in medical school, and my son, Misha, a chef, along with my nephew, Ben, and niece, Sarah, are so much of the reason I keep working to heal myself and the world.

And to my life partner and love, Brianna Welsh, who inspires me with her vision of a better world and helps me stay present to what really matters. Thank you for making my life brand-new again.

Glossary

amino acid: The chemical building block of proteins; the twenty essential amino acids that your body needs to build muscle all come from food, especially animal protein.

AMP: Adenosine monophosphate; ATP shares its energy in the body by giving one or two of its phosphate molecules to fuel cells, turning into adenosine di- or monophosphate (ADP or AMP).

AMPK: AMP-activated kinase, a nutrient-sensing system that detects dips in energy and turns on or off based on how much energy your body needs—a key longevity switch.

ATP: Adenosine triphosphate, the fuel your cells use to run everything. Your body creates ATP from burning calories and oxygen.

autophagy: The process of cellular recycling and renewal, key to life (and health) extension. It is the process of breaking down old proteins and molecules into their basic building blocks, allowing us to make new proteins and parts.

cell: The smallest structural unit of life; cells perform all the fundamental functions our bodies need to live.

chelation: Use of a binding agent to remove heavy metals from cells and tissues so they can be excreted in the urine or stool.

chromosomes: The structures that contain DNA and are held together by proteins. Human cells have 46 chromosomes, 23 from your mother and 23 from your father.

CRISPR: Gene-editing tool formally known as clustered regularly interspaced short palindromic repeats.

cytokines: Messengers of the immune system, or immune molecules.

DNA: Deoxyribonucleic acid, the molecule that encodes the information for your cells to function and replicate, aka your genetic code.

dysbiosis: The overgrowth of inflammatory bugs and depletion of anti-inflammatory bugs, driving leaky gut.

enzymes: Proteins made up of strings of amino acids that catalyze all the chemical reactions in your body.

epigenetics: A term that means "above the genome." It is the study of how your behaviors and environment create bookmarks on your genes, determining which genes are turned on or off.

epigenome: The sum of all the tags that modify the expression and function of the genome (genetic code). It regulates which genes are turned on or off. Think of the epigenome as the keystrokes on your computer keyboard, or the keys of a piano, that determine which instructions you give your computer or which song you play on the piano.

exosomes: Little packets of healing, anti-inflammatory, repair, and growth factors found inside stem cells.

exposome: The total of all the exposures (diet, lifestyle, toxins, stress, etc.) that influence your gene expression (mostly through epigenetics) and determine 90 percent of disease and aging.

gene: A specific sequence of DNA that codes for a specific protein.

genome: Your entire genetic blueprint or DNA.

heat shock proteins (HSPs): Healing proteins that help or recycle damaged proteins and activate antioxidant and repair systems.

hormesis: Good stress; a low level of biological adversity that stimulates repair in the body and improves the health and survival of cells.

immunome: The set of genes and proteins that constitute the immune system.

inflammaging: Systemic chronic inflammation that causes age-related disease.

metabolite: An intermediate or end product of metabolism that has various functions, including fuel, structure, signaling, and stimulatory and inhibitory effects on enzymes.

metabolome: The complete set of chemicals in your body. Many molecules in your metabolome are from your microbiome.

methylation: The process of adding or removing methyl groups (CH_3) that regulates energy production, gene expression, neurotransmitters, detoxification, and more. It is controlled by many enzymes dependent on vitamin B_{12} and B_6 and folate.

microbiome: The ecosystem of trillions of bugs that live in your digestive tract and on your skin and are intimately tied to every aspect of your health.

mitochondria: The powerhouse of cells where your energy (ATP, AMP) is made; mitochondria combine calories from food with oxygen and turn it into the energy needed to run everything in your body.

mTOR: Mammalian target of rapamycin, which is our built-in system for making new proteins and recycling old proteins through autophagy. The mTOR gene provides instructions for making the mTOR protein. This protein is found in various cell types throughout the body, including brain cells. mTOR regulates protein production, which influences cell growth, division, and survival. It is especially important for growth and development of the brain.

NAD+: Nicotinamide adenine dinucleotide, a chemical used in more than 500 chemical reactions in the body, including energy production and regulating sirtuin activity. Healthy eating and exercise raise NAD+ levels.

photobiomodulation: The use of long-wavelength infrared and red-light therapy to improve eyesight, cognitive ability and mobility, and skin aging.

phytochemicals: Beneficial medicinal molecules found in plants.

plasmapheresis: Transfer plasma exchange, a way to clean the blood. The process involves separating your white and red blood cells and platelets from the plasma and replacing the plasma with another form of protein such as albumin. Plasmapheresis is used in treating autoimmune disease and is being explored as a longevity treatment.

protein: A string of amino acids folded into a 3D structure. Each protein performs a specific role to help cells grow, divide, and function. All living things are made up of proteins, as well as carbohydrates, lipids (fats), and nucleic acids.

proteome: The entire complement of proteins that is or can be expressed by a cell, tissue, or organism.

rapamycin: A compound with immune-modulating functions in humans that may extend life span and improve health by inhibiting mTOR.

regenerative medicine: Emerging therapies to improve musculoskeletal-system function, to relieve pain without medication, and to regenerate health and promote longevity with stem cells, exosomes, peptides, ozone, natural killer cells, and plasmapheresis.

senescent cells (aka zombie cells): Normal cells that have stopped dividing, but start to release inflammatory molecules instead of dying. Zombie cells result from telomere shortening, DNA damage, and epigenetic changes.

senolytics: Natural and pharmaceutical compounds that can kill zombie cells, stop the progression of inflammaging, and allow for tissue repair, rejuvenation, and remodeling.

sirtuins: A family of signaling proteins that regulate aging and gene transcription (the making of new proteins), lower inflammation and oxidative stress, and improve metabolism and cellular energy production. Sirtuins are key players in the health and function of mitochondria, the heart of our metabolism.

stem cells: Cells with the potential to turn into a specialized cell, to divide into more stem cells, or to deliver healing and repair compounds to damaged cells and tissues. Most cells in your body already have specific roles and cannot become different kinds of cells.

telomeres: The protective end caps on chromosomes that shorten as we age. If they shorten too much, cells stop dividing (to create new cells) and can turn into senescent (zombie) cells.

transcriptome: The full range of messenger RNA (mRNA) molecules expressed by an organism. This is the mechanism by which our genes are "transcribed," or read, by the RNA.

Resources

Dr Mark Hyman's Websites

drhyman.com
functionhealth.com
gutfood.com
youngforeverbook.com/resources
store.drhyman.com for programs and supplements

The UltraWellness Center

55 Pittsfield Road, Suite 9
Lenox Commons
Lenox, MA 01240

If you'd like to book a virtual or in-person appointment with my clinic, visit ultrawellnesscenter.com or call (413) 637-9991.

The Cleveland Clinic Center for Functional Medicine

9500 Euclid Avenue/Q-2
Cleveland, OH 44195

If you'd like to book a virtual or in-person appointment with my clinic, visit my.clevelandclinic.org/departments/functional-medicine or call (216) 445-6900.

Functional Medicine

Find a functional medicine practitioner to guide you in the assessment, diagnosis, and treatment of your imbalances at the Institute for Functional Medicine (ifm.org).

Food Resources

Periodic Table of Food (foodperiodictable.org): a periodic table of the tens of thousands of potentially beneficial medicinal molecules called phytochemicals found in the plant kingdom.

Gut Food (gutfood.com): a multivitamin for daily gut support (soon to be available in the UK).

Pesticide Action Network (pan-uk.org): a source for information on toxic levels of pesticides on produce and toxins in personal-care products.

Clean Fish (cleanfish.com): a source to find fish that is sustainably harvested or farmed.

Hill Farm Real Food (hillfarmrealfood.co.uk): a source of A2 milk—a type of milk that has A2 casein, which is better tolerated than A1 casein, found in industrially raised cows. It has not been readily available in the UK since 2019 but can be obtained from some small suppliers.

Eversfield Organic (eversfieldorganic.co.uk) and Field and Flower (fieldandflower.co.uk): affordable grass-fed meat and safe fish.

Marine Stewardship Council (msc.org/uk): a great source of frozen and canned sustainably harvested wild fish with low levels of toxins.

Planet Organic (planetorganic.com): an online grocery store; a great source of healthy food and personal care and household cleaning products.

Primal Meats (primalmeats.co.uk): grass-fed meat and pasture-raised poultry.

Big Bold Health (bigboldhealth.com): a great source of Himalayan Tartary buckwheat flour (not currently available in the UK) and key supplements including HTB Rejuvenate and Dutch Harbor Omega.

Hormesis Therapies

Low-Oxygen Therapy

Cellgym (cellgym.com): a machine with a tight-fitting face mask that puts you through hypoxia and hyperoxia.

Hypoxia exercise masks from altitudeperformance.co.uk

Cold Therapy

The Plunge (thecoldplunge.com)

Saunas

Sunlighten Saunas (sunlighten.com)
Higher Dose sauna blanket (higherdose.com)

Home Ozone Therapy

Rectal ozone machine (simplyO3.com; pharmi-tech.co.uk)

Hyperbaric Oxygen Therapy

Oxygen Health Systems (oxygenhealthsystems.com) and Hyperbaric World Services (hyperbaricchambers.co.uk): sources for home machines.

Infrared and Red-Light Therapy

Joovv (joovv.com) and Red Light Therapy UK (red-light-therapy.co.uk)

Regenerative Medicine

Biorest Medical (bioresetinternational.com): Dr Matt Cook has established centers for regenerative medicine that treat a wide range of orthopedic, chronic pain, and chronic disease problems.

Hudson Medical and Wellness (hudsonmedical.com): Dr Jonathan Kuo and his team also established centers for regenerative medicine that treat a wide range of orthopedic, chronic pain, and chronic disease problems.

Sleep Aids

Smart light bulbs (bestreviews.com/home/light-bulbs/best-smart -light-bulb)
Blue-blocker glasses (truedark.com or boncharge.com)

Fitness

TB12 Sports (Tb12sports.com): former NFL player Tom Brady's program of band workouts and pliability.

Supplements

For a full list of longevity supplements and brands I recommend, go to youngforeverbook.com/resources.

BodyBio E-Lyte (bodybio.com)
Urolithin A from Mitopure (mitopure.com)
Gut Food (gutfood.com): soon to be available in the UK.

Trauma, Stress, and Relationships

Handel Group (Handelgroup.com): personal coaching. They also have a self-guided program called Inner.U.

Dynamic Neural Retraining System (retrainingthebrain.com): Dynamic Neural Retraining System helps regulate a mal-adapted stress response involved in many chronic illnesses, such as long COVID, chronic fatigue syndrome, multiple chemical sensitivity, fibromyalgia, chronic Lyme disease, food sensitivities, anxiety, chronic pain, postural orthostatic tachycardia syndrome, and others.

Pain Spa (painspa.co.uk): Stellate ganglion blocks (SGBs) to treat pain conditions driven by the sympathetic or stress response in the nervous system, such as stress, anxiety, PTSD, and depression.

MAPS (Multidisciplinary Association for Psychedelic Studies; maps .org): leading the way on research and FDA approval for use in mental health.

Quantified-Self Metrics

- Oura Ring (ouraring.com)
- Whoop (whoop.com)
- Fitbit (fitbit.com)

- Garmin Smart Watches (garmin.com)
- Apple Watch (apple.com)
- Eight Sleep (eightsleep.com)
- Levels Health for continuous glucose monitoring (sign up at levelshealth.com/hyman); not currently available in the UK. A similar system is available from FreeStyle Libre (freestylelibre. co.uk)

Testing

Function Health (functionhealth.com): a company that provides a simple way to get access to a complete set of over 100 lab tests at a low cost with periodic retesting every six to twelve months to measure your progress. Additional available tests include True Diagnostic DNA methylation and telomeres, iAge, Galleri cancer screening, and more. Use the promo code YOUNGFOR-EVER (not available in the UK) at functionhealth.com.

Scan.Com (uk.scan.com): a company that offers full-body MRI scans.

Functional Medicine Diagnostic Labs

ArminLabs (arminlabs.com)

Genova Labs (gdx.net)

Cyrex (cyrexlabs.com)

Doctor's Data (doctorsdata.com)

Nordic Labs for DNA testing (nordiclabs.com)

QuickSilver Scientific (quicksilverscientific.com)

MyMycoLab (mymycolab.com)

3X4 Genetics (3X4genetics.com; tests not available from the UK.)

Notes

INTRODUCTION

1. Healthy Aging Team. "The Top 10 Most Common Chronic Conditions in Older Adults." National Council on Aging. April 23, 2021. https://www.ncoa.org /article/the-top-10-most-common-chronic-conditions-in-older-adults.
2. "XT9T Ageing-Related." ICD-11 for Mortality and Morbidity Statistics, version 02/2022. https://icd.who.int/browse11/l-m/en#/http%3a%2f%2fid.who .int%2ficd%2fentity%2f459275392.
3. Steele A. *Ageless: The New Science of Getting Older without Getting Old.* New York: Anchor, 2021.
4. Goldman D. "The Economic Promise of Delayed Aging." *Cold Spring Harb Perspect Med.* 2015;6(2):a025072.

CHAPTER 1: The Quest for the Fountain of Youth

1. Fries JF. "Aging, Natural Death, and the Compression of Morbidity." *N Engl J Med.* 1980 Jul 17;303(3):130–35.
2. Hubert HB, Bloch DA, Oehlert JW, Fries JF. "Lifestyle Habits and Compression of Morbidity." *J Gerontol A Biol Sci Med Sci.* 2002 Jun;57(6):M347–51.
3. Knoops KT, et al. "Mediterranean Diet, Lifestyle Factors, and 10-Year Mortality in Elderly European Men and Women: The HALE Project." *JAMA.* 2004 Sep 22;292(12):1433–39.
4. Scott AJ, Ellison M, Sinclair DA. "The Economic Value of Targeting Aging." *Nat Aging.* 2021;1:616–23.
5. "Health and Economic Costs of Chronic Diseases." National Center for Chronic Disease Prevention and Health Promotion, Centers for Disease Control and Prevention. Last reviewed August 10, 2022. https://www.cdc.gov /chronicdisease/about/costs/index.htm.
6. Araújo J, Cai J, Stevens J. "Prevalence of Optimal Metabolic Health in American Adults: National Health and Nutrition Examination Survey 2009–2016." *Metab Syndr Relat Disord.* 2019 Feb;17(1):46–52.
7. O'Hearn M, Lauren BN, Wong JB, Kim DD, Mozaffarian D. "Trends and Disparities in Cardiometabolic Health among U.S. Adults, 1999–2018." *J Am Coll Cardiol.* 2022 Jul 12;80(2):138–51.

‎

8. O'Hearn M, Liu J, Cudhea F, Micha R, Mozaffarian D. "Coronavirus Disease 2019 Hospitalizations Attributable to Cardiometabolic Conditions in the United States: A Comparative Risk Assessment Analysis." *J Am Heart Assoc.* 2021 Feb;10(5):e019259.

9. Zolman ON. "Longevity Escape Velocity Medicine: A New Medical Specialty for Longevity?" *Rejuvenation Res.* 2018 Feb;21(1):1–2.

10. Davidsohn N, et al. "A Single Combination Gene Therapy Treats Multiple Age-Related Diseases." *Proc Natl Acad Sci U S A.* 2019 Nov 19;116(47):23505–11; Lu Y, et al. "Reprogramming to Recover Youthful Epigenetic Information and Restore Vision." *Nature.* 2020 Dec;588(7836):124–29; Jaijyan DK, et al. "New Intranasal and Injectable Gene Therapy for Healthy Life Extension." *Proc Natl Acad Sci U S A.* 2022 May 17;119(20): e2121499119.

11. Takahashi K, Yamanaka S. "Induction of Pluripotent Stem Cells from Mouse Embryonic and Adult Fibroblast Cultures by Defined Factors." *Cell.* 2006 Aug 25;126(4):663–76.

CHAPTER 2: The Root Causes of Aging

1. "Percent of U.S. Adults 55 and over with Chronic Conditions." National Center for Health Statistics, Centers for Disease Control and Prevention. November 6, 2015. Accessed July 28, 2022. https://www.cdc.gov/nchs/health_policy/adult_chronic_conditions.htm.

2. Wiertsema SP, van Bergenhenegouwen J, Garssen J, Knippels LM. "The Interplay between the Gut Microbiome and the Immune System in the Context of Infectious Diseases throughout Life and the Role of Nutrition in Optimizing Treatment Strategies." *Nutrients.* 2021;13(3):886. doi:10.3390/nu13030886.

CHAPTER 3: Biological versus Chronological Age

1. Horvath S, Raj K. "DNA Methylation-Based Biomarkers and the Epigenetic Clock Theory of Ageing." *Nat Rev Genet.* 2018 Jun;19(6):371–84.

2. Fitzgerald KN, Hodges R, Hanes D, et al. "Potential Reversal of Epigenetic Age Using a Diet and Lifestyle Intervention: A Pilot Randomized Clinical Trial." *Aging (Albany NY).* 2021 Apr 12;13(7):9419–32.

3. Moore S, et al. "Epigenetic Correlates of Neonatal Contact in Humans." *Dev Psychopathol.* 2017;29(5):1517–38.

4. Fujisawa TX, Nishitani S, Takiguchi S, Shimada K, Smith AK, Tomoda A. "Oxytocin Receptor DNA Methylation and Alterations of Brain Volumes in Maltreated Children." *Neuropsychopharmacol.* 2019 Nov;44(12):2045–53.

5. Bernal AJ, Jirtle RL. "Epigenomic Disruption: The Effects of Early Developmental Exposures." *Birth Defects Res A Clin Mol Teratol.* 2010;88(10):938–44.

6. Waterland R, Jirtle R. "Transposable Elements: Targets for Early Nutritional Effects on Epigenetic Gene Regulation." *Mol. Cell. Biol.* 2003;23(15):5293–

5300; Dolinoy DC, Wiedman J, Waterland R, Jirtle RL. "Maternal Genistein Alters Coat Color and Protects Avy Mouse Offspring from Obesity by Modifying the Fetal Epigenome." *Environ Health Perspect.* 2006;114(4): 567–572.

7. Rappaport SM. "Implications of the Exposome for Exposure Science." *J Expo Sci Environ Epidemiol.* 2011 Jan–Feb;21(1):5–9.

8. Youssef NA, Lockwood L, Su S, Hao G, Rutten BPF. "The Effects of Trauma, with or without PTSD, on the Transgenerational DNA Methylation Alterations in Human Offsprings." *Brain Sci.* 2018;8:83.

9. Van Cauwenbergh O, Di Serafino A, Tytgat J, Soubry A. "Transgenerational Epigenetic Effects from Male Exposure to Endocrine-Disrupting Compounds: A Systematic Review on Research in Mammals." *Clin Epigenetics.* 2020 May 12;12(1):65.

10. Fahy GM, Brooke RT, Watson JP, et al. "Reversal of Epigenetic Aging and Immunosenescent Trends in Humans." *Aging Cell.* 2019 Dec;18(6).

11. Chen L, Dong Y, Bhagatwala J, Raed A, Huang Y, Zhu H. "Effects of Vitamin D3 Supplementation on Epigenetic Aging in Overweight and Obese African Americans with Suboptimal Vitamin D Status: A Randomized Clinical Trial." *J Gerontol A Biol Sci Med Sci.* 2019;74(1):91–98.

12. Berendsen AAM, van de Rest O, Feskens EJM, et al. "Changes in Dietary Intake and Adherence to the NU-AGE Diet Following a One-Year Dietary Intervention among European Older Adults—Results of the NU-AGE Randomized Trial." *Nutrients.* 2018 Dec 4;10(12):1905.

13. Fitzgerald KN, Hodges R, Hanes D, et al. "Potential Reversal of Epigenetic Age Using a Diet and Lifestyle Intervention: A Pilot Randomized Clinical Trial." *Aging (Albany NY).* 2021 Apr 12;13(7):9419–32.

CHAPTER 4: The Ten Hallmarks of Aging

1. Konner M, Eaton SB. "Paleolithic Nutrition: Twenty-Five Years Later." *Nutr Clin Pract.* 2010 Dec;25(6):594–602; Carrera-Bastos P, Fontes-Villalba M, O'Keefe JH, Lindeberg S, Cordain L. "The Western Diet and Lifestyle and Diseases of Civilization." *Res. Rep. Clin. Cardiol.* 2011;2:15–35.

2. Zou Z, Tao T, Li H, Zhu X. "mTOR Signaling Pathway and mTOR Inhibitors in Cancer: Progress and Challenges." *Cell Biosci.* 2020 Mar 10;10:31.

3. Salminen A, Kaarniranta K. "AMP-Activated Protein Kinase (AMPK) Controls the Aging Process via an Integrated Signaling Network." *Ageing Res Rev.* 2012 Apr;11(2):230–41.

4. Kulkarni AS, Gubbi S, Barzilai N. "Benefits of Metformin in Attenuating the Hallmarks of Aging." *Cell Metab.* 2020 Jul 7;32(1):15–30.

5. Diabetes Prevention Program (DPP) Research Group. "The Diabetes Prevention Program (DPP): Description of Lifestyle Intervention." *Diabetes Care.* 2002;25(12):2165–71.

6. Ludwig DS, et al. "The Carbohydrate-Insulin Model: A Physiological Perspective on the Obesity Pandemic." *Am J Clin Nutr.* 2021 Sep 13;114(6): 1873–85.

7. McKenzie AL, et al. "Type 2 Diabetes Prevention Focused on Normalization of Glycemia: A Two-Year Pilot Study." *Nutrients.* 2021;13(3):749.

8. McKenzie AL, et al. "Type 2 Diabetes Prevention Focused on Normalization of Glycemia: A Two-Year Pilot Study." *Nutrients.* 2021;13(3):749.

9. Chung MY, Choi HK, Hwang JT. "AMPK Activity: A Primary Target for Diabetes Prevention with Therapeutic Phytochemicals." *Nutrients.* 2021 Nov 12;13(11):4050.

10. Imai S, Guarente L. "NAD+ and Sirtuins in Aging and Disease." *Trends Cell Biol.* 2014;24(8):464–71.

11. Grabowska W, Sikora E, Bielak-Zmijewska A. "Sirtuins, a Promising Target in Slowing Down the Ageing Process." *Biogerontology.* 2017;18(4):447–76.

12. Chen C, Zhou M, Ge Y, Wang X. "SIRT1 and Aging Related Signaling Pathways." *Mech Ageing Dev.* 2020 Apr;187:111215.

13. Lennerz B, Lennerz JK. "Food Addiction, High-Glycemic-Index Carbohydrates, and Obesity." *Clin Chem.* 2018 Jan;64(1):64–71.

14. The Periodic Table of Food Initiative. https://foodperiodictable.org.

15. Wątroba M, Dudek I, Skoda M, Stangret A, Rzodkiewicz P, Szukiewicz D. "Sirtuins, Epigenetics and Longevity." *Ageing Res Rev.* 2017 Nov;40:11–19.

16. Bertoldo MJ, Listijono DR, Ho WJ, et al. "NAD$^+$ Repletion Rescues Female Fertility during Reproductive Aging." *Cell Rep.* 2020 Feb 11;30(6):1670–81.e7.

17. Yoshino J, Baur JA, Imai SI. "NAD$^+$ Intermediates: The Biology and Therapeutic Potential of NMN and NR." *Cell Metab.* 2018 Mar 6;27(3):513–28.

18. Zhu Y, Tchkonia T, Pirtskhalava T, et al. "The Achilles' Heel of Senescent Cells: From Transcriptome to Senolytic Drugs." *Aging Cell.* 2015;14(4):644–58.

19. Araújo J, Cai J, Stevens J. "Prevalence of Optimal Metabolic Health in American Adults: National Health and Nutrition Examination Survey 2009–2016." *Metab Syndr Relat Disord.* 2019 Feb;17(1):46–52.

20. Burkitt DP. "Are Our Commonest Diseases Preventable?" *Prev Med.* 1977;6:556–59.

21. Quagliani D, Felt-Gunderson P. "Closing America's Fiber Intake Gap: Communication Strategies from a Food and Fiber Summit." *Am J Lifestyle Med.* 2016;11(1):80–85.

22. Coffin CS, Shaffer EA. "The Hot Air and Cold Facts of Dietary Fibre." *Can J Gastroenterol.* 2006;20(4):255–56.

23. Mowat AM. "Historical Perspective: Metchnikoff and the Intestinal Microbiome." *J Leukoc Biol.* 2021 Mar;109(3):513–17.

24. Wikoff WR, Anfora AT, Liu J, et al. "Metabolomics Analysis Reveals Large Effects of Gut Microflora on Mammalian Blood Metabolites." *Proc Natl Acad Sci U S A.* 2009 Mar 10;106(10):3698–703.

25. Wiciński M, Sawicka E, Gębalski J, Kubiak K, Malinowski B. "Human Milk Oligosaccharides: Health Benefits, Potential Applications in Infant Formulas, and Pharmacology." *Nutrients.* 2020;12(1):266.

26. Duranti S, Lugli GA, Mancabelli L, et al. "Prevalence of Antibiotic Resistance Genes among Human Gut-Derived Bifidobacteria." *Appl Environ Microbiol.* 2017;83:e02894-16.

27. Coman V, Vodnar DC. "Gut Microbiota and Old Age: Modulating Factors and Interventions for Healthy Longevity." *Exp Gerontol.* 2020 Nov;141:111095.

28. Fulop T, Larbi A, Pawelec G, et al. "Immunology of Aging: The Birth of Inflammaging." *Clin Rev Allergy Immunol.* 2021 Sep 18:1–14.

29. "84,000 Chemicals on the Market, Only 1% Have Been Tested for Safety." EcoWatch. July 6, 2015. https://www.ecowatch.com/84-000-chemicals-on-the-market-only-1-have-been-tested-for-safety-1882062458.html.

CHAPTER 5: Dying of Too Much or Too Little

1. Cordain L, et al. "Plant-Animal Subsistence Ratios and Macronutrient Energy Estimations in Worldwide Hunter-Gatherer Diets." *Am J Clin Nutr.* 2000;71: 682–92.

2. Galland L. "Diet and Inflammation." *Nutr Clin Pract.* 2010 Dec;25(6):634–40.

3. Malesza IJ, Malesza M, Walkowiak J, et al. "High-Fat, Western-Style Diet, Systemic Inflammation, and Gut Microbiota: A Narrative Review." *Cells.* 2021 Nov 14;10(11):3164.

4. GBD 2017 Diet Collaborators. "Health Effects of Dietary Risks in 195 Countries, 1990–2017: A Systematic Analysis for the Global Burden of Disease Study 2017." *Lancet.* 2019;393:1958–72.

5. "Noncommunicable Diseases." World Health Organization. April 13, 2021. https://www.who.int/news-room/fact-sheets/detail/noncommunicable-diseases.

6. Taubes G. *The Case Against Sugar.* New York: Knopf, 2016.

7. Schnabel L, et al. "Association between Ultraprocessed Food Consumption and Risk of Mortality among Middle-Aged Adults in France." *JAMA Intern Med.* 2019;179:490–98.

8. Martínez Steele E, et al. "Ultra-Processed Foods and Added Sugars in the US Diet: Evidence from a Nationally Representative Cross-Sectional Study." *BMJ Open.* 2016;6:e009892.

9. "Only 1 in 10 Adults Get Enough Fruits or Vegetables." Division of Nutrition, Physical Activity, and Obesity, Centers for Disease Control and Prevention. Last reviewed February 16, 2021. https://www.cdc.gov/nccdphp/dnpao/division-information/media-tools/adults-fruits-vegetables.html.

10. Franceschi C, Garagnani P, Vitale G, Capri M, Salvioli S. "Inflammaging and 'Garb-aging.'" *Trends Endocrinol Metab.* 2017;28:199–212.

11. Serhan CN, Levy BD. "Resolvins in Inflammation: Emergence of the Pro-Resolving Superfamily of Mediators." *J Clin Invest*. 2018;128:2657–69.
12. Muller DN, Wilck N, Haase S, Kleinewietfeld M, Linker RA. "Sodium in the Microenvironment Regulates Immune Responses and Tissue Homeostasis." *Nat Rev Immunol*. 2019;19:243–54.
13. Slavich GM, Cole SW. "The Emerging Field of Human Social Genomics." *Clin Psychol Sci*. 2013;1:331–48.
14. De la Iglesia HO, et al. "Ancestral Sleep." *Curr Biol*. 2016;26:R271–R272.
15. Raichlen DA, et al. "Physical Activity Patterns and Biomarkers of Cardiovascular Disease Risk in Hunter-Gatherers." *Am J Hum Biol*. 2017;29:e22919.
16. Blackwell DL, Clarke TC. "State Variation in Meeting the 2008 Federal Guidelines for Both Aerobic and Muscle-Strengthening Activities through Leisure-Time Physical Activity among Adults Aged 18–64: United States, 2010–2015." *Natl Health Stat Report*. 2018 Jun;112:1–22.
17. Ludwig DS, Ebbeling CB. "The Carbohydrate-Insulin Model of Obesity: Beyond 'Calories In, Calories Out.'" *JAMA Intern Med*. 2018;178(8):1098–1103.
18. Garatachea N, Pareja-Galeano H, Sanchis-Gomar F, et al. "Exercise Attenuates the Major Hallmarks of Aging." *Rejuvenation Res*. 2015;18(1):57–89.
19. Santos-Lozano A, et al. "Physical Activity and Alzheimer Disease: A Protective Association." *Mayo Clin Proc*. 2016;91:999–1020.
20. Hollar DW. "Biomarkers of Chondriome Topology and Function: Implications for the Extension of Healthy Aging." *Biogerontology*. 2017 Apr;18(2):201–15.
21. Ding D, Van Buskirk J, Nguyen B, et al. "Physical Activity, Diet Quality and All-Cause Cardiovascular Disease and Cancer Mortality: A Prospective Study of 346 627 UK Biobank Participants." *Br J Sports Med*. 2022 Jul 10:bjsports-2021-105195.
22. Leigh-Hunt N, Bagguley D, Bash K, et al. "An Overview of Systematic Reviews on the Public Health Consequences of Social Isolation and Loneliness." *Public Health*. 2017 Nov;152:157–71.
23. Flegal KM, Kit BK, Orpana H, Graubard BI. "Association of All-Cause Mortality with Overweight and Obesity Using Standard Body Mass Index Categories: A Systematic Review and Meta-Analysis." *JAMA*. 2013 Jan 2;309(1):71–82.
24. Lin J, Epel E. "Stress and Telomere Shortening: Insights from Cellular Mechanisms." *Ageing Res Rev*. 2022 Jan;73:101507.
25. Slavich GM, Cole SW. "The Emerging Field of Human Social Genomics." *Clin Psychol Sci*. 2013;1(3):331–48.
26. Steptoe A, Shankar A, Demakakos P, Wardle J. "Social Isolation, Loneliness, and All-Cause Mortality in Older Men and Women." *Proc Natl Acad Sci U S A*. 2013;110:5797–5801.

27. Rariden C, SmithBattle L, Yoo JH, Cibulka N, Loman D. "Screening for Adverse Childhood Experiences: Literature Review and Practice Implications." *J Nurse Pract.* 2021;17(1):98–104.

28. Hatori M, et al. "Global Rise of Potential Health Hazards Caused by Blue Light–Induced Circadian Disruption in Modern Aging Societies." *NPJ Aging Mech Dis.* 2017;3:9.

29. Irwin MR, Olmstead R, Carroll JE. "Sleep Disturbance, Sleep Duration, and Inflammation: A Systematic Review and Meta-Analysis of Cohort Studies and Experimental Sleep Deprivation." *Biol Psychiatry.* 2016 Jul 1;80(1):40–52.

30. Sengupta A, Weljie AM. "Metabolism of Sleep and Aging: Bridging the Gap Using Metabolomics." *Nutr Healthy Aging.* 2019 Dec 19;5(3):167–84.

31. Hatori M, et al. "Global Rise of Potential Health Hazards Caused by Blue Light–Induced Circadian Disruption in Modern Aging Societies." *NPJ Aging Mech Dis.* 2017;3:9.

32. Franceschi C, Garagnani P, Parini P, Giuliani C, Santoro A. "Inflammaging: A New Immune-Metabolic Viewpoint for Age-Related Diseases." *Nat Rev Endocrinol.* 2018;159:1–15.

33. DeJong EN, Surette MG, Bowdish DME. "The Gut Microbiota and Unhealthy Aging: Disentangling Cause from Consequence." *Cell Host Microbe.* 2020 Aug 12;28(2):180–89.

34. Rook G, Bäckhed F, Levin BR, McFall-Ngai MJ, McLean AR. "Evolution, Human-Microbe Interactions, and Life History Plasticity." *Lancet.* 2017;390: 521–30.

35. Sturgeon C, Fasano A. "Zonulin, a Regulator of Epithelial and Endothelial Barrier Functions, and Its Involvement in Chronic Inflammatory Diseases." *Tissue Barriers.* 2016;4:e1251384.

36. Qi Y, et al. "Intestinal Permeability Biomarker Zonulin Is Elevated in Healthy Aging." *J Am Med Direc Assoc.* 2017;18:810.e1–810.e4.

37. Sturgeon C, Fasano A. "Zonulin, a Regulator of Epithelial and Endothelial Barrier Functions, and Its Involvement in Chronic Inflammatory Diseases." *Tissue Barriers.* 2016;4(4).

38. Pawelec G, et al. "Human Immunosenescence: Is It Infectious?" *Immunol Rev.* 2005;205:257–68.

39. Rook G, Bäckhed F, Levin BR, McFall-Ngai MJ, McLean AR. "Evolution, Human-Microbe Interactions, and Life History Plasticity." *Lancet.* 2017;390: 521–30.

40. Sly PD, et al. "Health Consequences of Environmental Exposures: Causal Thinking in Global Environmental Epidemiology." *Ann Glob Health.* 2016; 82:3–9.

41. "Body Burden: The Pollution in Newborns." Environmental Working Group. July 14, 2005. https://www.ewg.org/research/body-burden-pollution-newborns.

CHAPTER 6: Foundations of Longevity

1. Parker A, et al. "Fecal Microbiota Transfer between Young and Aged Mice Reverses Hallmarks of the Aging Gut, Eye, and Brain." *Microbiome.* 2022 Apr 29;10(1):68.
2. Gomaa EZ. "Human Gut Microbiota/Microbiome in Health and Diseases: A Review." *Antonie Van Leeuwenhoek.* 2020 Dec;113(12):2019–40.
3. Evangelou E, Ntritsos G, Chondrogiorgi M, et al. "Exposure to Pesticides and Diabetes: A Systematic Review and Meta-Analysis." *Environ Int.* 2016;91:60–68.
4. Navas-Acien A, Guallar E, Silbergeld EK, Rothenberg SJ. "Lead Exposure and Cardiovascular Disease—a Systematic Review." *Environ Health Perspect.* 2007;115(3):472–82.
5. Yusuf S, et al. "INTERHEART Study Investigators. Effect of Potentially Modifiable Risk Factors Associated with Myocardial Infarction in 52 Countries (the INTERHEART Study): Case-Control Study." *Lancet.* 2004 Sep 11–17;364(9438):937–52.
6. Araújo J, Cai J, Stevens J. "Prevalence of Optimal Metabolic Health in American Adults: National Health and Nutrition Examination Survey 2009–2016." *Metab Syndr Relat Disord.* 2019 Feb;17(1):46–52.
7. Berrazaga I, Micard V, Gueugneau M, Walrand S. "The Role of the Anabolic Properties of Plant- versus Animal-Based Protein Sources in Supporting Muscle Mass Maintenance: A Critical Review." *Nutrients.* 2019;11(8):1825.
8. Van Vliet S, Burd NA, van Loon LJ. "The Skeletal Muscle Anabolic Response to Plant- versus Animal-Based Protein Consumption." *J Nutr.* 2015;145(9):1981–91.

CHAPTER 7: Eating for Longevity

1. Barnett JA, Gibson DL. "Separating the Empirical Wheat from the Pseudoscientific Chaff: A Critical Review of the Literature Surrounding Glyphosate, Dysbiosis and Wheat-Sensitivity." *Front Microbiol.* 2020 Sep 25;11:556729.
2. "National Health and Nutrition Examination Survey: 2013–2014 Data Documentation, Codebook, and Frequencies: Glyphosate (GLYP)—Urine (SSGLYP_H)." June 2022. https://wwwn.cdc.gov/Nchs/Nhanes/2013-2014/SSGLYP_H.htm.
3. Singer-Englar T, Barlow G, Mathur R. "Obesity, Diabetes, and the Gut Microbiome: An Updated Review." *Expert Rev Gastroenterol Hepatol.* 2019;13(1):3–15.
4. Lerner A, Matthias T. "Changes in Intestinal Tight Junction Permeability Associated with Industrial Food Additives Explain the Rising Incidence of Autoimmune Disease." *Autoimmun Rev.* 2015;14(6):479–89.
5. Routy B, et al. "Gut Microbiome Influences Efficacy of PD-1-Based Immunotherapy Against Epithelial Tumors." *Science.* 2018 Jan 5;359(6371):91–97.
6. Innes JK, Calder PC. "Omega-6 Fatty Acids and Inflammation." *Prostaglandins Leukot Essent Fatty Acids.* 2018;132:41–48.

7. Li Z, Henning SM, Zhang Y, et al. "Antioxidant-Rich Spice Added to Hamburger Meat during Cooking Results in Reduced Meat, Plasma, and Urine Malondialdehyde Concentrations." *Am J Clin Nutr.* 2010;91(5):1180–84.

8. Ames BN. "A Role for Supplements in Optimizing Health: The Metabolic Tune-Up." *Arch Biochem Biophys.* 2004;423(1):227–34.

9. Ames BN. "The Metabolic Tune-Up: Metabolic Harmony and Disease Prevention." *J Nutr.* 2003;133(5 Suppl 1):1544S–1548S.

10. "Chemical Cuisine Ratings." Center for Science in the Public Interest. https://www.cspinet.org/page/chemical-cuisine-ratings.

11. Joe B, Vijaykumar M, Lokesh BR. "Biological Properties of Curcumin—Cellular and Molecular Mechanisms of Action." *Crit Rev Food Sci Nutr.* 2004;44(2):97–111.

12. Roberts CK, Barnard RJ, Sindhu RK, Jurczak M, Ehdaie A, Vaziri ND. "A High-Fat, Refined-Carbohydrate Diet Induces Endothelial Dysfunction and Oxidant/Antioxidant Imbalance and Depresses NOS Protein Expression." *J Appl Physiol (1985).* 2005;98(1):203–10.

13. Barringer TA, Hacher L, Sasser HC. "Potential Benefits on Impairment of Endothelial Function after a High-Fat Meal of 4 Weeks of Flavonoid Supplementation." *Evid Based Complement Alternat Med.* 2011;2011:796958.

14. Neri S, Signorelli SS, Torrisi B, et al. "Effects of Antioxidant Supplementation on Postprandial Oxidative Stress and Endothelial Dysfunction: A Single-Blind, 15-Day Clinical Trial in Patients with Untreated Type 2 Diabetes, Subjects with Impaired Glucose Tolerance, and Healthy Controls." *Clin Ther.* 2005;27(11):1764–73.

15. Van Bussel BC, Henry RM, Ferreira I, et al. "A Healthy Diet Is Associated with Less Endothelial Dysfunction and Less Low-Grade Inflammation over a 7-Year Period in Adults at Risk of Cardiovascular Disease." *J Nutr.* 2015;145(3):532–40.

16. Zehr KR, Walker MK. "Omega-3 Polyunsaturated Fatty Acids Improve Endothelial Function in Humans at Risk for Atherosclerosis: A Review." *Prostaglandins Other Lipid Mediat.* 2018;134:131–40.

17. Schwingshackl L, Christoph M, Hoffmann G. "Effects of Olive Oil on Markers of Inflammation and Endothelial Function—A Systematic Review and Meta-Analysis." *Nutrients.* 2015 Sep 11;7(9):7651–75. doi:10.3390/nu7095356.

18. Uwitonze AM, Razzaque MS. "Role of Magnesium in Vitamin D Activation and Function." *J Am Osteopath Assoc.* 2018;118(3):181–89.

19. Rosenberg A, Mangialasche F, Ngandu T, Solomon A, Kivipelto M. "Multidomain Interventions to Prevent Cognitive Impairment, Alzheimer's Disease, and Dementia: From FINGER to World-Wide FINGERS." *J Prev Alzheimers Dis.* 2020;7(1):29–36; Isaacson RS, et al. "Individualized Clinical Management of Patients at Risk for Alzheimer's Dementia." *Alzheimers Dement.* 2019 Dec;15(12):1588–1602.

20. Broom GM, Shaw IC, Rucklidge JJ. "The Ketogenic Diet as a Potential Treat-ment and Prevention Strategy for Alzheimer's Disease." *Nutrition.* 2019 Apr;60:118–21.

21. Norwitz NG, Dalai SS, Palmer CM. "Ketogenic Diet as a Metabolic Treatment for Mental Illness." *Curr Opin Endocrinol Diabetes Obes.* 2020 Oct;27(5):269–74.

22. Dean OM, Hodge AM, Berk M. "A Randomised Controlled Trial of Dietary Improvement for Adults with Major Depression (the 'SMILES' trial)." *BMC Med.* 2017 Jan 30;15(1):23. doi: 10.1186/s12916-017-0791-y. Erratum in *BMC Med.* 2018 Dec 28;16(1):236.

23. Berrazaga I, Micard V, Gueugneau M, Walrand S. "The Role of the Anabolic Properties of Plant- versus Animal-Based Protein Sources in Supporting Mus-cle Mass Maintenance: A Critical Review." *Nutrients.* 2019;11(8):1825.

24. Van Vliet S, Burd NA, van Loon LJ. "The Skeletal Muscle Anabolic Response to Plant- versus Animal-Based Protein Consumption." *J Nutr.* 2015;145(9):1981–91.

25. Brandt K, Mølgaard JP. "Organic Agriculture: Does It Enhance or Reduce the Nutritional Value of Plant Foods?" *J Sci Food Agric.* 2001;81:924–31.

26. Martel J, Ojcius DM, Ko YF, et al. "Hormetic Effects of Phytochemicals on Health and Longevity." *Trends Endocrinol Metab.* 2019 Jun;30(6):335–46.

27. Ping Z, et al. "Sulforaphane Protects Brains against Hypoxic-Ischemic Injury through Induction of Nrf2-Dependent Phase 2 Enzyme." *Brain Res.* 2010;1343: 178–85.

28. Han J, et al. "Epigallocatechin Gallate Protects against Cerebral Ischemia-Induced Oxidative Stress via Nrf2/ARE Signaling." *Neurochem Res.* 2014;39: 1292–99.

29. Eisenberg T, et al. "Cardioprotection and Lifespan Extension by the Natural Polyamine Spermidine." *Nat Med.* 2016;22:1428–38.

30. Malerba S, et al. "A Meta-Analysis of Prospective Studies of Coffee Consump-tion and Mortality for All Causes, Cancers and Cardiovascular Diseases." *Eur J Epidemiol.* 2013;28:527–39.

31. Martucci M, et al. "Mediterranean Diet and Inflammaging within the Hor-mesis Paradigm." *Nutr Rev.* 2017;75:442–55.

32. Luthar Z, Golob A, Germ M, Vombergar B, Kreft I. "Tartary Buckwheat in Human Nutrition." *Plants (Basel).* 2021 Apr 5;10(4):700.

33. Mayorov V, Uchakin P, Amarnath V, et al. "Targeting of Reactive Isolevug-landins in Mitochondrial Dysfunction and Inflammation." *Redox Biol.* 2019 Sep;26:101300.

34. Anhe FF, et al. "A Polyphenol-Rich Cranberry Extract Protects from Diet-Induced Obesity, Insulin Resistance and Intestinal Inflammation in Associa-tion with Increased *Akkermansia* spp. Population in the Gut Microbiota of Mice." *Gut.* 2015;64:872–83.

35. Singh A, D'Amico D, Andreux PA, et al. "Urolithin A Improves Muscle Strength, Exercise Performance, and Biomarkers of Mitochondrial Health in a

Randomized Trial in Middle-Aged Adults." *Cell Rep Med.* 2022 May 17;3(5):100633.

36. Strasser B, Volaklis K, Fuchs D, Burtscher M. "Role of Dietary Protein and Muscular Fitness on Longevity and Aging." *Aging Dis.* 2018 Feb 1;9(1):119–32.

37. Bauer J, et al. "Evidence-Based Recommendations for Optimal Dietary Protein Intake in Older People: A Position Paper from the PROT-AGE Study Group." *J Am Med Dir Assoc.* 2013 Aug;14(8):542–59.

CHAPTER 8: Moving for Longevity

1. Gremeaux V, Gayda M, Lepers R, Sosner P, Juneau M, Nigam A. "Exercise and Longevity." *Maturitas.* 2012 Dec;73(4):312–17.

2. Piercy KL, Troiano RP, Ballard RM, et al. "The Physical Activity Guidelines for Americans." *JAMA.* 2018 Nov 20;320(19):2020–28.

3. Saint-Maurice PF, Graubard BI, Troiano RP, et al. "Estimated Number of Deaths Prevented through Increased Physical Activity among US Adults." *JAMA Intern Med.* 2022;182(3):349–52.

4. Mailing LJ, Allen JM, Buford TW, Fields CJ, Woods JA. "Exercise and the Gut Microbiome." *Exerc Sport Sci Rev.* 2019;47(2):75–85. doi:10.1249/jes.00000000 00000183; Ticinesi A, Lauretani F, Tana C, Nouvenne A, Ridolo E, Meschi T. "Exercise and Immune System as Modulators of Intestinal Microbiome: Implications for the Gut-Muscle Axis Hypothesis." *Exerc Immunol Rev.* 2019;25:84–95.

5. Suzuki K. "Chronic Inflammation as an Immunological Abnormality and Effectiveness of Exercise." *Biomolecules.* 2019;9(6):223. doi:10.3390/biom9060223.

6. Huertas JR, Casuso RA, Agustín PH, Cogliati S. "Stay Fit, Stay Young: Mitochondria in Movement: The Role of Exercise in the New Mitochondrial Paradigm." *Oxid Med Cell Longev.* 2019;2019:1–18. doi:10.1155/2019/7058350; Hood DA, Memme JM, Oliveira AN, Triolo M. "Maintenance of Skeletal Muscle Mitochondria in Health, Exercise, and Aging." *Annu Rev Physiol.* 2019;81(1):19–41. doi:10.1146/annurev-physiol-020518-114310.

7. Hackney AC, Davis HC, Lane AR. "Growth-Hormone-Insulin-Like Growth Factor Axis, Thyroid Axis, Prolactin, and Exercise." *Sports Endocrinology.* Frontiers of Hormone Research. Basel: Karger; 2016:1–11. doi:10.1159/00044514; Hackney AC, Lane AR. "Exercise and the Regulation of Endocrine Hormones." *Molecular and Cellular Regulation of Adaptation to Exercise.* Progress in Molecular Biology and Translational Science. Waltham, MA: Academic Press; 2015:293–311.

8. Aguirre LE, Villareal DT. "Physical Exercise as Therapy for Frailty." *Frailty: Pathophysiology, Phenotype and Patient Care.* Nestlé Nutrition Institute Workshop Series. Basel: Karger; 2015:83–92. doi:10.1159/000382065; Mendonca GV, Pezarat-Correia P, Vaz JR, Silva L, Almeida ID, Heffernan KS. "Impact of Exercise Training on Physiological Measures of Physical Fitness in the Elderly." *Curr Aging Sci.* 2016;9(4):240–59.

9. Khazaee-Pool M, Sadeghi R, Majlessi F, Foroushani AR. "Effects of Physical Exercise Programme on Happiness among Older People." *J Psychiatr Ment Health Nurs.* 2014;22(1):47–57; Forbes H, Fichera E, Rogers A, Sutton M. "The Effects of Exercise and Relaxation on Health and Wellbeing." *Health Econ.* 2017;26(12). doi:10.1002/hec.3477; Ruegsegger GN, Booth FW. "Health Benefits of Exercise." *Cold Spring Harbor Perspectives in Medicine.* 2018. Accessed July 22, 2020. http://perspectivesinmedicine.cshlp.org/content/8/7/a029694.long.

10. Nomikos NN, Nikolaidis PT, Sousa CV, Papalois AE, Rosemann T, Knechtle B. "Exercise, Telomeres, and Cancer: 'The Exercise-Telomere Hypothesis.'" *Front Physiol.* 2018;9. doi:10.3389/fphys.2018.01798; Arsenis NC, You T, Ogawa EF, Tinsley GM, Zuo L. "Physical Activity and Telomere Length: Impact of Aging and Potential Mechanisms of Action." *Oncotarget.* 2017 Jul 4;8(27):45008–19; Lin X, Zhou J, Dong B. "Effect of Different Levels of Exercise on Telomere Length: A Systematic Review and Meta-Analysis." *J Rehabil Med.* 2019;51(7):473–78.

11. Miyamoto L. "AMPK as a Metabolic Intersection between Diet and Physical Exercise." *Yakugaku Zasshi.* 2018;138(10):1291–96. doi:10.1248/yakushi.18 -00091-6; Hoffman NJ, Parker BL, Chaudhuri R, et al. "Global Phosphoproteomic Analysis of Human Skeletal Muscle Reveals a Network of Exercise -Regulated Kinases and AMPK Substrates." *Cell Metab.* 2015;22(5):922–35.

12. Vargas-Ortiz K, Pérez-Vázquez V, Macías-Cervantes MH. "Exercise and Sirtuins: A Way to Mitochondrial Health in Skeletal Muscle." *Int J Mol Sci.* 2019;20(11):2717.

13. Mazucanti C, Cabral-Costa J, Vasconcelos A, Andreotti D, Scavone C, Kawamoto E. "Longevity Pathways (mTOR, SIRT, Insulin/IGF-1) as Key Modulatory Targets on Aging and Neurodegeneration." *Curr Top Med Chem.* 2015;15(21):2116–38. doi:10.2174/1568026615666615061012571; Gremeaux V, Gayda M, Lepers R, Sosner P, Juneau M, Nigam A. "Exercise and Longevity." *Maturitas.* 2012;73(4):312–17. doi:10.1016/j.maturitas.2012.09.012; Zhao M, Veeranki SP, Magnussen CG, Xi B. "Recommended Physical Activity and All-Cause and Cause Specific Mortality in US Adults: Prospective Cohort Study." *BMJ.* July 2020:m2031. doi:10.1136/bmj.m2031.

14. Gielen S, Laughlin MH, O'Conner C, Duncker DJ. "Exercise Training in Patients with Heart Disease: Review of Beneficial Effects and Clinical Recommendations." *Prog Cardiovasc Dis.* 2015;57(4):347–55; Bove AA. "Exercise and Heart Disease." *Methodist DeBakey Cardiovasc J.* 2016;12(2):74–75. Moraes-Silva IC, Rodrigues B, Coelho-Junior HJ, Feriani DJ, Irigoyen M-C. "Myocardial Infarction and Exercise Training: Evidence from Basic Science." *Exercise for Cardiovascular Disease Prevention and Treatment.* Advances in Experimental Medicine and Biology. Singapore: Springer; 2017:139–53.

15. Stout NL, Baima J, Swisher AK, Winters-Stone KM, Welsh J. "A Systematic Review of Exercise Systematic Reviews in the Cancer Literature (2005–

2017)." *PM R.* 2017;9. doi:10.1016/j.pmrj.2017.07.074; Idorn M, Straten PT. "Exercise and Cancer: From 'Healthy' to 'Therapeutic'?" *Cancer Immunol Immunother.* 2017;66(5):667–71. doi:10.1007/s00262-017-1985-z.

16. Kirwan JP, Sacks J, Nieuwoudt S. "The Essential Role of Exercise in the Management of Type 2 Diabetes." *Cleve Clin J Med.* 2017;84(7 suppl 1). doi:10.3949/ccjm.84.s1.03; Balducci S, Sacchetti M, Haxhi J, et al. "Physical Exercise as Therapy for Type 2 Diabetes Mellitus." *Diabetes Metab Res Rev.* 2014;30(S1):13–23. doi:10.1002/dmrr.2514; Karstoft K, Pedersen BK. "Exercise and Type 2 Diabetes: Focus on Metabolism and Inflammation." *Immunol Cell Biol.* 2015;94(2):146–50. doi:10.1038/icb.2015.101; Hamasaki H. "Interval Exercise Therapy for Type 2 Diabetes." *Curr Diabetes Rev.* 2018;14(2):129–37. doi:10.2174/1573399812666161101103655; Borghouts LB, Keizer HA. "Exercise and Insulin Sensitivity: A Review." *Int J Sports Med.* 2000;21(1):1–12. doi:10.1055/s-2000-8847.

17. Marshall RN, Smeuninx B, Morgan PT, Breen L. "Nutritional Strategies to Offset Disuse-Induced Skeletal Muscle Atrophy and Anabolic Resistance in Older Adults: From Whole-Foods to Isolated Ingredients." *Nutrients.* 2020;12(5):1533.

CHAPTER 9: Optimizing Your Lifestyle for Longevity

1. Biber DD, Ellis R. "The Effect of Self-Compassion on the Self-Regulation of Health Behaviors: A Systematic Review." *J Health Psychol.* 2017;24(14):2060–71. doi:10.1177/1359105317713361; Brown L, Bryant C, Brown V, Bei B, Judd F. "Self-Compassion, Attitudes to Ageing and Indicators of Health and Well-Being among Midlife Women." *Aging Ment Health.* 2015;20(10):1035–43. doi:10.1080/13607863.2015.1060946.

2. Dunne S, Sheffield D, Chilcot J. "Brief Report: Self-Compassion, Physical Health and the Mediating Role of Health-Promoting Behaviours." *J Health Psychol.* 2016;23(7):993–99. doi:10.1177/1359105316643377.

3. Friis AM, Consedine NS, Johnson MH. "Does Kindness Matter? Diabetes, Depression, and Self-Compassion: A Selective Review and Research Agenda." *Diabetes Spectr.* 2015;28(4):252–57. doi:10.2337/diaspect.28.4.252; Ferrari M, Cin MD, Steele M. "Self-Compassion Is Associated with Optimum Self-Care Behaviour, Medical Outcomes and Psychological Well-Being in a Cross-Sectional Sample of Adults with Diabetes." *Diabet Med.* 2017;34(11):1546–53. doi:10.1111/dme.13451.

4. Alizadeh S, Khanahmadi S, Vedadhir A, Barjasteh S. "The Relationship between Resilience with Self-Compassion, Social Support and Sense of Belonging in Women with Breast Cancer." *Asian Pac J Cancer Prev.* 2018;19(9):2469–74. doi:10.22034/APJCP.2018.19.9.2469.

5. Yang YC, Boen C, Gerken K, Li T, Schorpp K, Harris KM. "Social Relationships and Physiological Determinants of Longevity across the Human Life Span." *Proc Natl Acad Sci U S A.* 2016;113(3):578–83. doi:10.1073/pnas.1511085112.

6. Penzel IB, Persich MR, Boyd RL, Robinson MD. "Linguistic Evidence for the Failure Mindset as a Predictor of Life Span Longevity." *Ann Behav Med.* 2017;51(3):348–55. doi:10.1007/s12160-016-9857-x; Watkins ER. "Constructive and Unconstructive Repetitive Thought." *Psychol Bull.* 2008;134(2):163–206. doi:10.1037/0033-2909.134.2.163.

7. Gabrian M, Dutt AJ, Wahl H-W. "Subjective Time Perceptions and Aging Well: A Review of Concepts and Empirical Research—A Mini-Review." *Gerontology.* 2017;63(4):350–58. doi:10.1159/000470906.

8. Windsor TD, Curtis RG, Luszcz MA. "Sense of Purpose as a Psychological Resource for Aging Well." *Dev Psychol.* 2015;51(7):975–86. doi:10.1037/dev0000023.

9. Boccardi M, Boccardi V. "Psychological Wellbeing and Healthy Aging: Focus on Telomeres." *Geriatrics.* 2019;4(1):25. doi:10.3390/geriatrics4010025.

10. Epel ES, Blackburn EH, Lin J, et al. "Accelerated Telomere Shortening in Response to Life Stress." *Proc Natl Acad Sci U S A.* 2004;101(49):17312–15. doi:10.1073/pnas.0407162101.

11. Dunne S, Sheffield D, Chilcot J. "Brief Report: Self-Compassion, Physical Health and the Mediating Role of Health-Promoting Behaviours." *J Health Psychol.* 2016;23(7):993–99. doi:10.1177/1359105316643377.

12. Institute of Medicine (US) Committee on Sleep Medicine and Research. *Sleep Disorders and Sleep Deprivation: An Unmet Public Health Problem.* Colten HR, Altevogt BM, editors. Washington, DC: National Academies Press; 2006.

13. Mazzotti DR, Guindalini C, Moraes WA, et al. "Human Longevity Is Associated with Regular Sleep Patterns, Maintenance of Slow Wave Sleep, and Favorable Lipid Profile." *Front Aging Neurosci.* 2014;6:134.

14. Alimujiang A, Wiensch A, Boss J, et al. "Association Between Life Purpose and Mortality among US Adults Older Than 50 Years." *JAMA Netw Open.* 2019;2(5):e194270.

CHAPTER 10: Hormesis

1. Das SK, Balasubramanian P, Weerasekara YK. "Nutrition Modulation of Human Aging: The Calorie Restriction Paradigm." *Mol Cell Endocrinol.* 2017 Nov 5;455:148–57.

2. Rattan SI. "Hormetic Modulation of Aging and Longevity by Mild Heat Stress." *Dose Response.* 2006 May 22;3(4):533–46.

3. Laukkanen T, Khan H, Zaccardi F, Laukkanen JA. "Association between Sauna Bathing and Fatal Cardiovascular and All-Cause Mortality Events." *JAMA Intern Med.* 2015;175(4):542–48.

4. Laukkanen T, Kunutsor S, Kauhanen J, Laukkanen JA. "Sauna Bathing Is Inversely Associated with Dementia and Alzheimer's Disease in Middle-Aged Finnish Men." *Age Ageing.* 2017;46:245–49.

5. Knechtle B, Waśkiewicz Z, Sousa CV, Hill L, Nikolaidis PT. "Cold Water Swimming—Benefits and Risks: A Narrative Review." *Int J Environ Res Public Health.* 2020 Dec 2;17(23):8984.

6. Warburton DER, Bredin SSD. "Health Benefits of Physical Activity." *Curr Opin Cardiol.* 2017 Sep;32(5):541–56.

7. Mandsager K, Harb S, Cremer P, Phelan D, Nissen SE, Jaber W. "Association of Cardiorespiratory Fitness with Long-Term Mortality among Adults Undergoing Exercise Treadmill Testing." *JAMA Netw Open.* 2018;1(6):e183605.

8. Shen J, Tower J. "Effects of Light on Aging and Longevity." *Ageing Res Rev.* 2019;53:100913.

9. Stevens RG, Brainard GC, Blask DE, et al. "Adverse Health Effects of Nighttime Lighting: Comments on American Medical Association Policy Statement." *Am J Prev Med.* 201345(3):343–46.

10. Hamblin MR. "Mechanisms and Applications of the Anti-Inflammatory Effects of Photobiomodulation." *AIMS Biophys.* 2017;4(3):337–61; Weinrich TW, Coyne A, Salt TE, et al. "Improving Mitochondrial Function Significantly Reduces Metabolic, Visual, Motor and Cognitive Decline in Aged Drosophila melanogaster." *Neurobiol Aging.* 2017;60:34–43.

11. Glass GE. "Photobiomodulation: The Clinical Applications of Low-Level Light Therapy." *Aesthet Surg J.* 2021 May 18;41(6):723–38.

12. Bocci V, Zanardi I, Travagli V. "Potentiality of Oxygen-Ozonetherapy to Improve the Health of Aging People." *Curr Aging Sci.* 2010 Dec;3(3):177–87.

13. Bocci V. *Ozone: A New Medical Drug.* Dordrecht: Springer; 2011.

14. "WFOT's Review on Evidence Based Ozone Therapy." WFOT Scientific Advisory Committee 2015. https://www.wfoot.org/wp-content/uploads/2016/01/WFOT-OZONE-2015-ENG.pdf; Jacobs M-T. "Untersuchung uber Zwischenfalle und typische Komplikationen in der OzonSauerstoff-Therapie." *OzoNachrichten.* 1982;1:5.

15. Smith NL, Wilson AL, Gandhi J, Vatsia S, Khan SA. "Ozone Therapy: An Overview of Pharmacodynamics, Current Research, and Clinical Utility." *Med Gas Res.* 2017 Oct 17;7(3):212–19.

16. Elvis AM, Ekta JS. "Ozone Therapy: A Clinical Review." *J Nat Sci Biol Med.* 2011;2(1):66–70.

17. Hachmo Y, et al. "Hyperbaric Oxygen Therapy Increases Telomere Length and Decreases Immunosenescence in Isolated Blood Cells: A Prospective Trial." *Aging (Albany NY).* 2020 Nov 18;12(22):22445–56.

18. Hadanny A, Efrati S. "The Hyperoxic-Hypoxic Paradox." *Biomolecules.* 2020 Jun 25;10(6):958.

19. Li Y, Wang MS, Otecko NO, et al. "Hypoxia Potentially Promotes Tibetan Longevity." *Cell Res.* 2017;27(2):302–5. doi:10.1038/cr.2016.105.

20. Keane M, et al. "Insights into the Evolution of Longevity from the Bowhead Whale Genome." *Cell Rep.* 2015 Jan 6;10(1):112–22.

21. Yeo EJ. "Hypoxia and Aging." *Exp. Mol. Med.* 2019;51:1–15.
22. Serebrovska TV, et al. "Intermittent Hypoxia Training in Prediabetes Patients: Beneficial Effects on Glucose Homeostasis, Hypoxia Tolerance and Gene Expression." *Exp Biol Med (Maywood).* 2017 Sep;242(15):1542–52.
23. Serebrovska ZO, et al. "Intermittent Hypoxia-Hyperoxia Training Improves Cognitive Function and Decreases Circulating Biomarkers of Alzheimer's Disease in Patients with Mild Cognitive Impairment: A Pilot Study." *Int J Mol Sci.* 2019 Oct 30;20(21):5405.
24. Brown RP, Gerbarg PL. "Yoga Breathing, Meditation, and Longevity." *Ann N Y Acad Sci.* 2009 Aug;1172:54–62.

CHAPTER 11: Advanced Longevity Innovations

1. Scott AJ, Ellison M, Sinclair DA. "The Economic Value of Targeting Aging." *Nat Aging.* 2021;1:616–23.
2. Simpson DJ, Olova NN, Chandra T. "Cellular Reprogramming and Epigenetic Rejuvenation." *Clin Epigenetics.* 2021 Sep 6;13(1):170.
3. Zhu Y, Ge J, Huang C, Liu H, Jiang H. "Application of Mesenchymal Stem Cell Therapy for Aging Frailty: From Mechanisms to Therapeutics." *Theranostics.* 2021 Mar 31;11(12):5675–85. doi:10.7150/thno.46436.
4. Schulman IH, Balkan W, Hare JM. "Mesenchymal Stem Cell Therapy for Aging Frailty." *Front Nutr.* 2018 Nov 15;5:108.
5. Malek A, Bersinger NA. "Human Placental Stem Cells: Biomedical Potential and Clinical Relevance." *J Stem Cells.* 2011;6(2):75–92.
6. Hamdan Y, Mazini L, Malka G. "Exosomes and Micro-RNAs in Aging Process." *Biomedicines.* 2021;9(8):968.
7. Gurunathan S, Kang MH, Kim JH. "A Comprehensive Review on Factors Influences Biogenesis, Functions, Therapeutic and Clinical Implications of Exosomes." *Int J Nanomedicine.* 2021;16:1281–1312.
8. Gurunathan S, et al. "Review of the Isolation, Characterization, Biological Function, and Multifarious Therapeutic Approaches of Exosomes." *Cells.* 2019;8(4):307.
9. Apostolopoulos V, et al. "A Global Review on Short Peptides: Frontiers and Perspectives." *Molecules (Basel, Switzerland).* 2021 Jan 15;26(2):430.
10. Lau JL, Dunn MK. "Therapeutic Peptides: Historical Perspectives, Current Development Trends, and Future Directions." *Bioorg Med Chem.* 2018 Jun 1;26(10):2700–2707.
11. Thorner MO, Chapman IM, Gaylinn BD, Pezzoli SS, Hartman ML. "Growth Hormone-Releasing Hormone and Growth Hormone-Releasing Peptide as Therapeutic Agents to Enhance Growth Hormone Secretion in Disease and Aging." *Recent Prog Horm Res.* 1997;52:215–44; discussion 244–46.

12. Lau JL, Dunn MK. "Therapeutic Peptides: Historical Perspectives, Current Development Trends, and Future Directions." *Bioorg Med Chem.* 2018 Jun 1;26(10):2700–2707.
13. Becker PSA, et al. "Selection and Expansion of Natural Killer Cells for NK Cell-Based Immunotherapy." *Cancer Immunol Immunother.* 2016;65(4):477–84.
14. Du N, Guo F, Wang Y, Cui J. "NK Cell Therapy: A Rising Star in Cancer Treatment." *Cancers (Basel).* 2021 Aug 17;13(16):4129.
15. Tarazona R, Lopez-Sejas N, Guerrero B, et al. "Current Progress in NK Cell Biology and NK Cell-Based Cancer Immunotherapy." *Cancer Immunol Immunother.* 2020 May;69(5):879–99.
16. Pfeffer M, et al. "A Randomized, Controlled Clinical Trial of Plasma Exchange with Albumin Replacement for Alzheimer's Disease: Primary Results of the AMBAR Study." *Alzheimers Dement.* 2020 Oct;16(10):1412–25.
17. Kiprov DD, et al. "Case Report: Therapeutic and Immunomodulatory Effects of Plasmapheresis in Long-Haul COVID." *F1000Res.* 2021 Nov 24;10:1189.
18. Mehdipour M, et al. "Rejuvenation of Three Germ Layers Tissues by Exchanging Old Blood Plasma with Saline-Albumin." *Aging (Albany NY).* 2020 May 30;12(10):8790–819.
19. Roy A, Mantay M, Brannan C, Griffiths S. "Placental Tissues as Biomaterials in Regenerative Medicine." *BioMed Research International.* 2022;2022:1–26. doi:10.1155/2022/6751456.
20. Courseault J, Kessler E, Moran A, Labbe A. "Fascial Hydrodissection for Chronic Hamstring Injury." *Curr Sports Med Rep.* 2019 Nov;18(11):416–20.
21. Yamada S, Behfar A, Terzic A. "Regenerative Medicine Clinical Readiness." *Regen Med.* 2021;16(3):309–22.
22. Shallenberger F. "Prolozone™—Regenerating Joints and Eliminating Pain." *J Prolotherapy.* 2011;3(2):630–38. https://journalofprolotherapy.com/prolozone-regenerating-joints-and-eliminating-pain/.

CHAPTER 13: Testing

1. Nakhleh MK, et al. "Diagnosis and Classification of 17 Diseases from 1404 Subjects via Pattern Analysis of Exhaled Molecules." *ACS Nano.* 2017 Jan 24;11(1):112–25.
2. Navas-Acien A, Guallar E, Silbergeld EK, Rothenberg SJ. "Lead Exposure and Cardiovascular Disease—a Systematic Review." *Environ Health Perspect.* 2007;115(3):472–82.
3. Arshad T, Golabi P, Henry L, Younossi ZM. "Epidemiology of Non-Alcoholic Fatty Liver Disease in North America." *Curr Pharm Des.* 2020;26(10):993–97.
4. "Perceived Stress Scale." State of New Hampshire Employee Assistance Program. https://www.das.nh.gov/wellness/docs/percieved%20stress%20scale.pdf.

5. Sayed N, Huang Y, Nguyen K, et al. "An Inflammatory Aging Clock (iAge) Based on Deep Learning Tracks Multimorbidity, Immunosenescence, Frailty and Cardiovascular Aging." *Nat Aging*. 2021 Jul;1:598–615.

6. Hackshaw A, Clarke CA, Hartman AR. "New Genomic Technologies for Multi-Cancer Early Detection: Rethinking the Scope of Cancer Screening." *Cancer Cell*. 2022 Feb 14;40(2):109–13.

CHAPTER 14: Food as Medicine

1. Khaw K-T, Sharp SJ, Finikarides L, et al. "Randomised Trial of Coconut Oil, Olive Oil or Butter on Blood Lipids and Other Cardiovascular Risk Factors in Healthy Men and Women." *BMJ Open*. 2018;8(3). doi:10.1136/bmjopen-2017 -020167.

2. Higdon J. "Carotenoids." Linus Pauling Institute. January 1, 2020. Accessed July 22, 2020. https://lpi.oregonstate.edu/mic/dietary-factors/phytochemicals /carotenoids.

3. Yang P-M, Wu Z-Z, Zhang Y-Q, Wung B-S. "Lycopene Inhibits ICAM-1 Expression and NF-κB Activation by Nrf2-Regulated Cell Redox State in Human Retinal Pigment Epithelial Cells." *Life Sciences*. 2016;155:94–101. doi:10.1016/j.lfs.2016.05.006.

4. Higdon, J. "Carotenoids." Linus Pauling Institute. January 1, 2020. Accessed July 22, 2020. https://lpi.oregonstate.edu/mic/dietary-factors/phytochemicals /carotenoids.

5. Amalraj A, Pius A, Gopi S, Gopi S. "Biological Activities of Curcuminoids, Other Biomolecules from Turmeric and Their Derivatives—a Review." *J Tradit Complement Med*. 2017;7(2):205–33. doi:10.1016/j.jtcme.2016.05.005.

6. Higdon J. "Isothiocyanates." Linus Pauling Institute. January 1, 2020. Accessed July 22, 2020. https://lpi.oregonstate.edu/mic/dietary-factors/phytochemicals /isothiocyanates; Higdon J. "Indole-3-Carbinol." Linus Pauling Institute. January 1, 2020. Accessed July 22, 2020. https://lpi.oregonstate.edu/mic/dietary -factors/phytochemicals/indole-3-carbinol; Marcus JB. *Aging, Nutrition and Taste: Nutrition, Food Science and Culinary Perspectives for Aging Tastefully*. London: Academic Press; 2019.

7. Kim JK, Park SU. "Current Potential Health Benefits of Sulforaphane." *EXCLI Journal*. 2016;15:571–77. doi:10.17179/excli2016-485.

8. Khoo HE, Azlan A, Tang ST, Lim SM. "Anthocyanidins and Anthocyanins: Colored Pigments as Food, Pharmaceutical Ingredients, and the Potential Health Benefits." *Food Nutr Res*. 2017;61(1):1361779. doi:10.1080/16546628.20 17.1361779.

9. Magrone T, Russo MA, Jirillo E. "Cocoa and Dark Chocolate Polyphenols: From Biology to Clinical Applications." *Front Immunol*. 2017;8:677. doi:10.3389/ fimmu.2017.00677.

10. Khan N, Syed DN, Ahmad N, Mukhtar H. "Fisetin: A Dietary Antioxidant for Health Promotion." *Antioxid Redox Signal.* 2013;19(2):151–62. doi:10.1089/ars.2012.4901; Xu D, Hu M-J, Wang Y-Q, Cui Y-L. "Antioxidant Activities of Quercetin and Its Complexes for Medicinal Application." *Molecules.* 2019;24(6):1123. doi:10.3390/molecules24061123.

11. Salehi B, Venditti A, Sharifi-Rad M, et al. "The Therapeutic Potential of Apigenin." *Int J Mol Sci.* 2019;20(6):1305. doi:10.3390/ijms20061305.

12. Muhammad T, Ikram M, Ullah R, Rehman S, Kim M. "Hesperetin, a Citrus Flavonoid, Attenuates LPS-Induced Neuroinflammation, Apoptosis and Memory Impairments by Modulating TLR4/NF-κB Signaling." *Nutrients.* 2019;11(3): 648. doi:10.3390/nu11030648.

13. Spagnuolo C, Russo GL, Orhan IE, et al. "Genistein and Cancer: Current Status, Challenges, and Future Directions." *Adv Nutr.* 2015;6(4):408–19. doi:10.3945/an.114.008052.

14. van Lith R, Ameer GA. "Antioxidant Polymers as Biomaterial." In Dziubla T, Butterfield DA, eds. *Oxidative Stress and Biomaterials.* Waltham, MA: Academic Press; 2016:251–96.

15. Kozarski M, Klaus A, Jakovljevic D, et al. "Antioxidants of Edible Mushrooms." *Molecules.* 2015;20(10):19489–525. doi:10.3390/molecules201019489; Lu C-C, Hsu Y-J, Chang C-J, et al. "Immunomodulatory Properties of Medicinal Mushrooms: Differential Effects of Water and Ethanol Extracts on NK Cell-Mediated Cytotoxicity." *Innate Immun.* 2016;22(7):522–33. doi:10.1177/1753425916661402.

16. Sun W, Frost B, Liu J. "Oleuropein, Unexpected Benefits!" *Oncotarget.* 2017;8(11):17409. doi:10.18632/oncotarget.15538; Shamshoum H, Vlavcheski F, Tsiani E. "Anticancer Effects of Oleuropein." *BioFactors.* 2017;43(4):517–28. doi:10.1002/biof.1366; Ahamad J, Toufeeq I, Khan MA, et al. "Oleuropein: A Natural Antioxidant Molecule in the Treatment of Metabolic Syndrome." *Phytother Res.* 2019;33(12):3112–3128. doi:10.1002/ptr.6511.

17. Nishimura Y, Moriyama M, Kawabe K, et al. "Lauric Acid Alleviates Neuroinflammatory Responses by Activated Microglia: Involvement of the GPR40-Dependent Pathway." *Neurochem Res.* 2018;43(9):1723–35. doi:10.1007/s11064-018-2587-7; Nonaka Y, Takagi T, Inai M, et al. "Lauric Acid Stimulates Ketone Body Production in the KT-5 Astrocyte Cell Line." *J Oleo Sci.* 2016;65(8):693–99. doi:10.5650/jos.ess16069; Matsue M, Mori Y, Nagase S, et al. "Measuring the Antimicrobial Activity of Lauric Acid against Various Bacteria in Human Gut Microbiota Using a New Method." *Cell Transplant.* 2019;28(12):1528–41. doi:10.1177/0963689719881366.

18. Yang H, Shan W, Zhu F, Wu J, Wang Q. "Ketone Bodies in Neurological Diseases: Focus on Neuroprotection and Underlying Mechanisms." *Front Neurol.* 2019;10. doi:10.3389/fneur.2019.00585; Belluzzi A, Boschi S, Brignola C,

Munarini A, Cariani G, Miglio F. "Polyunsaturated Fatty Acids and Inflammatory Bowel Disease." *Am J Clin Nutr.* 2000;71(1 Suppl):339S–342S; Chowdhury R, Warnakula S, Kunutsor S, et al. "Association of Dietary, Circulating, and Supplement Fatty Acids with Coronary Risk: A Systematic Review and Meta-Analysis." *Ann Intern Med.* 2014;160(6):398–406.

19. Dorling JL, Martin CK, Redman LM. "Calorie Restriction for Enhanced Longevity: The Role of Novel Dietary Strategies in the Present Obesogenic Environment." *Ageing Res Rev.* 2020;64:101038.

20. Brandhorst S, Longo VD. "Protein Quantity and Source, Fasting-Mimicking Diets, and Longevity." *Adv Nutr.* 2019 Nov 1;10(Suppl 4):S340–S350.

21. Wei M, Longo VD, et. al. "Fasting-Mimicking Diet and Markers/Risk Factors for Aging, Diabetes, Cancer, and Cardiovascular Disease." *Sci Transl Med.* 2017 Feb 15;9(377):eaai8700.

22. Testa G, Biasi F, Poli G, Chiarpotto E. "Calorie Restriction and Dietary Restriction Mimetics: A Strategy for Improving Healthy Aging and Longevity." *Curr Pharm Des.* 2014;20(18):2950–77.

CHAPTER 15: The Young Forever Supplements for Longevity

1. Heaney R. "Long Latency Deficiency Diseases: Insights from Calcium and Vitamin D." *Am J Clin Nutr.* 2003;78:912–19.

2. "National Health and Nutrition Examination Survey," National Center for Health Statistics, Centers for Disease Control and Prevention. https://www.cdc.gov/nchs/nhanes/.

3. Uwitonze AM, Razzaque MS. "Role of Magnesium in Vitamin D Activation and Function." *J Am Osteopath Assoc.* 2018;118(3).

4. Pencina K, et al. "MIB-626, an Oral Formulation of a Microcrystalline Unique Polymorph of β-Nicotinamide Mononucleotide, Increases Circulating Nicotinamide Adenine Dinucleotide and Its Metabolome in Middle-aged and Older Adults." *J Gerontol A Biol Sci Med Sci.* 2022 Feb 19:glac049.

5. Yousefzadeh MJ, et al. "Fisetin Is a Senotherapeutic That Extends Health and Lifespan." *EBioMedicine.* 2018 Oct;36:18–28.

6. McCormack D, McFadden D. "A Review of Pterostilbene Antioxidant Activity and Disease Modification." *Oxid Med Cell Longev.* 2013;2013:575482.

7. Plotkin DL, Delcastillo K, Van Every DW, Tipton KD, Aragon AA, Schoenfeld BJ. "Isolated Leucine and Branched-Chain Amino Acid Supplementation for Enhancing Muscular Strength and Hypertrophy: A Narrative Review." *Int J Sport Nutr Exerc Metab.* 2021 May 1;31(3):292–301.

8. Dolan E, Artioli GG, Pereira RMR, Gualano B. "Muscular Atrophy and Sarcopenia in the Elderly: Is There a Role for Creatine Supplementation?" *Biomolecules.* 2019 Oct 23;9(11):642.

9. Padmavathi G, Roy NK, Bordoloi D, et al. "Butein in Health and Disease: A Comprehensive Review." *Phytomedicine.* 2017 Feb 15;25:118–27.

CHAPTER 16: The Young Forever Lifestyle Practices

1. Van der Ploeg HP, Chey T, Ding D, Chau JY, Stamatakis E, Bauman AE. "Standing Time and All-Cause Mortality in a Large Cohort of Australian Adults." *Prev Med.* 2014 Dec;69:187–91.
2. Allen J, Morelli V. "Aging and Exercise." *Clin Geriatr Med.* 2011 Nov;27(4): 661–71.
3. Madhivanan P, Krupp K, Waechter R, Shidhaye R. "Yoga for Healthy Aging: Science or Hype?" *Adv Geriatr Med Res.* 2021;3(3):e210016.
4. Smyth JM, Stone AA, Hurewitz A, Kaell A. "Effects of Writing about Stressful Experiences on Symptom Reduction in Patients with Asthma or Rheumatoid Arthritis: A Randomized Trial." *JAMA.* 1999;281(14):1304–9.
5. Deslandes A, Moraes H, Ferreira C, et al. "Exercise and Mental Health: Many Reasons to Move." *Neuropsychobiology.* 2009;59(4):191–98. doi:10.1159/000223730.
6. Vingren JL, Kraemer WJ, Ratamess NA, Anderson JM, Volek JS, Maresh CM. "Testosterone Physiology in Resistance Exercise and Training." *Sports Med.* 2010;40(12):1037–53. doi:10.2165/11536910-000000000-00000.
7. Lee MB, Hill CM, Bitto A, Kaeberlein M. "Antiaging Diets: Separating Fact from Fiction." *Science.* 2021 Nov 19;374(6570):eabe7365.
8. Strasser B, Burtscher M. "Survival of the Fittest: VO$_2$ max, a Key Predictor of Longevity?" *Front Biosci (Landmark Ed).* 2018 Mar 1;23(8):1505–16.

CHAPTER 17: The Young Forever Plan to Optimize Your Seven Core Biological Systems

1. Cattel F, Giordano S, Bertiond C, et al. "Ozone Therapy in COVID-19: A Narrative Review." *Virus Res.* 2021 Jan 2;291:198207.
2. Ibelli T, Templeton S, Levi-Polyachenko N. "Progress on Utilizing Hyperthermia for Mitigating Bacterial Infections." *Int J Hyperthermia.* 2018 Mar;34(2):144–56.
3. Cheng Y, Weng S, Yu L, Zhu N, Yang M, Yuan Y. "The Role of Hyperthermia in the Multidisciplinary Treatment of Malignant Tumors." *Integr Cancer Ther.* 2019 Jan–Dec;18:1534735419876345.
4. Gurunathan S, Kang MH, Kim JH. "A Comprehensive Review on Factors Influences Biogenesis, Functions, Therapeutic and Clinical Implications of Exosomes." *Int J Nanomedicine.* 2021;16:1281–312.
5. Meeusen R, van der Veen P, Joos E, Roeykens J, Bossuyt A, De Meirleir K. "The Influence of Cold and Compression on Lymph Flow at the Ankle." *Clin J Sport Med.* 1998 Oct;8(4):266–71.

6. Shallenberger F. "Prolozone™—Regenerating Joints and Eliminating Pain." *J Prolotherapy.* 2011;3(2):630–38. https://journalofprolotherapy.com/prolozone-regenerating-joints-and-eliminating-pain/.

7. Zanos P, Gould TD. "Mechanisms of Ketamine Action as an Antidepressant." *Mol Psychiatry.* 2018 Apr;23(4):801–11.

8. Olmsted KL, et al. "Effect of Stellate Ganglion Block Treatment on Posttraumatic Stress Disorder Symptoms: A Randomized Clinical Trial." *JAMA Psychiatry.* 2020 Feb 1;77(2):130–38.

9. Luoma JB, Chwyl C, Bathje GJ, Davis AK, Lancelotta R. "A Meta-Analysis of Placebo-Controlled Trials of Psychedelic-Assisted Therapy." *J Psychoactive Drugs.* 2020 Sep–Oct;52(4):289–99.

10. Winkelman M. "Psychedelics as Medicines for Substance Abuse Rehabilitation: Evaluating Treatments with LSD, Peyote, Ibogaine and Ayahuasca." *Curr Drug Abuse Rev.* 2014;7(2):101–16.

Index

About the Author

Dr Mark Hyman believes that we all deserve a life of vitality—and that we have the potential to create it for ourselves. That's why he is dedicated to tackling the root causes of chronic disease by harnessing the power of functional medicine to transform health care.

Dr Hyman and his team work every day to empower people, organizations, and communities to heal their bodies and minds and to improve our social and economic resilience. Dr Hyman is a practicing family physician, a fourteen-time *New York Times* bestselling author, and an internationally recognized leader, speaker, educator, and advocate in his field. His podcast, *The Doctor's Farmacy,* is one of the top 100 of all podcasts, with more than 150 million downloads. He is the founder and senior adviser of the Cleveland Clinic Center for Functional Medicine. He is also the founder and medical director of The UltraWellness Center, board president for clinical affairs of the Institute for Functional Medicine, and a regular medical contributor on many television shows and networks, including *CBS This Morning, Today, Good Morning America,* CNN, and *The View.*

His nonprofit, the Food Fix Campaign, is dedicated to transforming the dysfunctional policies that shape our food and agricultural systems. The Food Fix Campaign has played a key role in supporting the first White House Conference on Hunger, Nutrition, and Health and creating the first federal entity dedicated to addressing chronic disease and nutrition through updating and coordinating all food programs and policies. Their work has supported $20 billion in federal funding for regenerative agriculture.

Dr Hyman works with individuals and organizations as well as policy makers and influencers. He has testified before both the White

House Commission on Complementary and Alternative Medicine and the Senate Working Group on Health Care Reform on Functional Medicine. He has consulted with the surgeon general on diabetes prevention and participated in the 2009 White House Forum on Prevention and Wellness. Senator Tom Harkin of Iowa nominated Dr Hyman for the President's Advisory Group on Prevention, Health Promotion, and Integrative and Public Health. In addition, Dr Hyman has worked with President Bill Clinton, presenting at the Clinton Foundation's Health Matters, Achieving Wellness in Every Generation conference, and the Clinton Global Initiative, as well as with the World Economic Forum on global health issues. He is a winner of the Linus Pauling Award, the Nantucket Project Award, and the Christian Book of the Year Award for *The Daniel Plan,* and was inducted into the Books for Better Life Hall of Fame.

Dr Hyman also works with fellow leaders in his field to help people and communities thrive—with Rick Warren, Dr Mehmet Oz, and Dr Daniel Amen, he created the Daniel Plan, a faith-based initiative that helped the Saddleback Church collectively lose 250,000 pounds. With Dr Dean Ornish and Dr Michael Roizen, Dr Hyman crafted and helped introduce the Take Back Your Health Act of 2009 to the United States Senate to provide for reimbursement of lifestyle treatment of chronic disease. And with Tim Ryan in 2015, he helped introduce the ENRICH Act into Congress to fund nutrition in medical education. Dr Hyman plays a substantial role in a major film produced by Laurie David and Katie Couric, released in 2014, called *Fed Up,* which addresses childhood obesity, and in *Kiss the Ground* and other many other health-focused documentaries. Please join him in helping us all take back our health at www.drhyman.com, or follow him on Twitter, Facebook, and Instagram (@drmarkhyman).

yellow
kite

books to help you live a good life

Join the conversation and tell
us how you live a #goodlife

𝕏 @yellowkitebooks
f YellowKiteBooks
𝒫 Yellow Kite Books
📷 YellowKiteBooks